A Nutritional Approa
www.Livin

LIVING F(

The Amazing Stories of 11 People Who Beat Disease Using Raw & Whole Foods

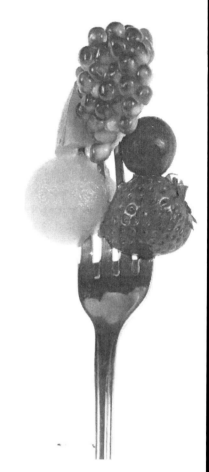

"Cancer, Lupus, Arthritis, Bi-Polar, Multiple Sclerosis & More ... Gone"

-- Living Food Reporter

www.LivingFoodCures.com

Living Food Cures: The Amazing Stories of 11 People Who Beat Disease Using Raw & Whole Foods

Published by BookSpecs Publishing
16 Sunset Ave
Pennsville, NJ 08070
www.LivingFoodCures.com

ISBN 978-0-9721461-2-8
LCCN 2009905723

This book is available as a product for both affiliate selling and also as a product for special joint ventures with entrepreneurs, booksellers and/or blog owners in the food and health information industry. Visit www.LivingFoodCures.com and contact the author for more information about how you can sell it.

Acknowledgments

A number of individuals significantly contributed to this work. Each one of them has my sincere appreciation and thanks for their unique contributions.

First, special acknowledgement is reserved for those who willingly offered some of their time and personal information by letting me interview them. They shared details from events that took place during difficult periods in their lives.

These individuals also gave some incredibly helpful tips out of their stories of healing for readers who are now facing similar obstacles and health challenges. Their testimonials about how consuming raw and whole foods can impact health were inspiring to me personally, and will also be fascinating to anyone who reads this book with an open mind. They are (in order of appearance): Larry Jones, Justin Gingerella, Judy Livingstone, Karen Hood, Suzy Hoseus, Lee Jernigan, Faye Lambeth, Mariana Pina-Bergtold, Danny Garris, Jerrod Sessler, and Samuel Ericsson.

Additional thanks goes to Julie Wilkins, whose interview is featured in a downloadable "bonus chapter" to this book, which you may download at the Internet webpage address given after the Table of Contents.

When I first decided to write this book I knew I wanted to fill it with testimonies from those who've personally experienced the kind of healing that can come through a fundamental diet change. After all, what better way to validate the teaching that consuming mostly raw vegetables, fruits, nuts and small portions of cooked whole foods can allow the body to heal itself?

One of the best places to find great healing testimonials was from a Christian-based health organization called Hallelujah Acres. Its founder, Rev. George Malkmus, began

Hallelujah Acres back around 1990 in order to take his message about diet and healing to a broad audience.

Their magazine back then was called, "Back to the Garden." My mother-in-law gave me this publication to read one afternoon back in the early 90s. It introduced me to the idea that living foods can often bring levels of physical healing from diseases that most people would consider incredible.

As I hope you will see, anyone might find himself or herself discovering this truth, regardless of their religious views, after speaking with people who have similar testimonies of dramatic wellness after changing to a plant-based diet. Not everyone who was interviewed or quoted within this book is a Christian. But they all seem to express ideas about food, nutrition and health that are very similar to the general theme of this book.

It also seems clear to me that the folks at Hallelujah Acres discovered a combination of dietary elements that have helped untold numbers of people get well who were once sick. It's important to acknowledge this book probably would never have been written if I hadn't read their publications years ago. Any individuals who obtained wellness simply incorporated sound information they had read about into their own lives.

Tim and Anita Koch, who run a Hallelujah Acres Lifestyle Center in North Carolina, were particularly helpful in connecting me with several of those who share their story of healing in this book. You can visit **www.whollyalive.com** to find out more about them and their unique work in helping others.

Finally, Nancy Bubeck spent many hours reviewing this material when it was still in manuscript form. And Eleanor Roper created the book cover. Eleanor and her husband Robert are both skilled artists within the publishing industry. See **www.RobertRoper.com** for more details and contact information.

Your Free Audio Gift ...

How to Change to a Living Foods Diet ... Without Going Totally Nuts ☺

This FREE audio (available in mp3 format) features the Living Food Reporter and a special guest talking about how to transition to a living foods diet. Whether fighting disease, or pursuing optimal health, there is nothing that beats mostly raw foods. **Topics include:**

- What are the major obstacles to changing to a healthy diet (and how to overcome them)

- The most important foods in a healing diet (and what foods to avoid consuming too much of)

- 3 Ways to organize your kitchen for quick meal preparation

- How to prepare basic foods easily (Great meals don't have to be a chore)

- Where to buy produce at the best rates. (Some tips on locating choice food sellers in your area)

- Why eating raw can actually be LESS expensive than a Standard American Diet

- What is "detoxification" ... and how might it impact your diet change?

- Techniques for getting over unhealthy food cravings

- Plus other living food tips ...

To download your free audio now go to:
www.LivingFoodCures.com/Book/Free-Book-Audio.html

Table of Contents

Introduction

The premise of this book is fairly simple. Consuming the right kinds of foods and shunning the wrong ones can pave the way to health and possibly even help the body heal itself from chronic, severe or debilitating diseases.

The title of this book, "*Living Food Cures*," doesn't mean food itself brings direct healing. It means the right foods offer your body the materials it needs for incredible self-healing properties to function at peak performance.

Many people would probably say this idea, in and of itself, sounds reasonable to some extent. But most people have no idea how powerful this concept actually is. Nor do most individuals know the full extent to which thousands of people have applied it to find relief from pain, suffering, debilitating conditions and even escape the clutches of physical death itself.

Living foods enable your body's God-given immune system to function at an incredibly high level. They also provide the building blocks required for healthy new cells to replace diseased or dying ones in the body's constant cell-regeneration process.

Nutritional cure or healing isn't direct -- it's indirect. Food isn't medicine per se. But as you'll soon see, it may be better than medicine at certain times.

While the exact proportions of how these foods are consumed may be a little different among those who've experienced dramatic health recovery, the general rule is that the more food consumed in raw form the better. One facet of this is that foods taken ripe from the garden always offer higher nutritional content than processed foods. And raw foods that were grown organically are best.

If you're open to this idea then it's not hard to understand why many raw-foodists have experienced miraculous healing in their bodies simply by changing their diet. It also becomes easy to understand why many people in the "whole foods" and "macrobiotic" food communities have experienced similar health results.

The biggest key to approaching diet as a vehicle for health seems to be the avoidance of animal-based products in favor of plant-based food products. When plant-based foods are consumed in a state that is as unprocessed, or "natural" as possible, then incredible things can happen if either a sick person is trying to get well or a healthy person is trying to enjoy optimal health.

This is often the case even when an individual doesn't embrace 100% veganism.[1] Many practitioners of a macrobiotic diet[2] approach, for example, consume very few animal-based products in favor of mostly whole foods and high quantities of raw vegetables and fruits. That is often enough to enable recovery from serious illness.

The point here is that there are common "raw food factors" associated with diet and healing. By covering them I'll end up sharing what I think is the "best" nutritional approach to health and wellness. This book, however, isn't the final word. As a matter of fact, it may not even be my final word on the subject. It reflects my current understanding of things based upon my research up to the time of this publication.

Important Note: Regardless of what you may read someone else has done, you should NEVER stop taking prescribed medications except under the care of your own physician. To simply stop taking certain medications could result in death or severe injury. You should always consult with your own physician before attempting to stop taking any prescribed medicines.

As you read through this book you may get the impression I'm always against "conventional medicine." That isn't true. But as you will see in some of these stories, it may be appropriate to ask yourself whether always relying upon conventional medicine is the single best approach to eliminating disease and experiencing bodily healing.

Questions can be asked about conventional medicine in the same way that skeptics would question a nutritional attempt at healing. For example: Is it wrong for a sick patient to ask their doctor whether or not taking medications to simply mask symptoms is a path towards true healing? Is devastating chemotherapy good medicine considering how sick many patients get when undergoing it? Does it make sense to try experimental drugs if a proven nutritional approach to healing hasn't been tried first?

Such questions are worth asking. Are they not?

Each and every day, doctors inform tens of thousands of people across the globe that they've been diagnosed with a severe illness. For many individuals hearing this news means their life will never be the same again. For some, the consequence of receiving such a report could mean the beginning of the end of their physical life.

If you or a loved one has received a gloomy report from a doctor then you know how fear and uncertainty can quickly invade your life. This book is written to encourage either you or someone you know if serious chronic disease is now creating a health challenge. And if you wish to prevent serious illness then the message contained within these pages just may keep you from ever having to battle a debilitating or terminal illness.

Does this sound too good to be true? It might. I certainly thought so about 15 years ago ... when I first heard stories like the ones you're about to read.

11

1

Can a Change in Diet Allow
the Body to Heal Itself?

Disease happens inside the human body for various reasons. There are causes for disease. Is there anything that can be done to help the body remedy these causes so it can begin healing? Yes.

The human body can often rid itself of much disease ... in an almost miraculous way. If you (or a loved one) are now battling disease then there is hope for you in the same way there was hope for those featured in this book.

Somewhere back in the mid-1990s, my mother-in-law came to our house for a visit. She set a magazine in front of me about health and nutrition and said she was amazed by its contents, especially the testimonials. Apparently, individuals in the magazine claimed they were totally healed from all types of diseases, including things like cancer, diabetes, lupus and severe arthritis ... after simply changing their diet.

"*Uh Huh*," I thought to myself. "*Sure they were. It's nothing more than quackery, except this form of delusion was coming under the guise of nutrition instead of some 'magic potion' sold inside a bottle.*"

Since I'd always thought myself to be a healthy eater I perused the reading material out of curiosity ... especially the stories. What I read almost seemed fictional, especially considering the severity of the diseases, depth of sicknesses and reported miraculous healings.

There were some things within the material, however, that seemed plausible. For instance, the notion a person's immune system could be suppressed because of poor nutrition, which could then lead to sickness.

Accepting that idea, however, opened the door for more questions: Could a proper diet cause a person's immune system to begin functioning at an optimal level? Could the diseased condition then be reversed if it were brought about by poor nutrition or a suppressed immune system?

My initial skepticism about the material was taken over by thoughts of theoretical plausibility. The stories in the magazine certainly conveyed a hint of truthfulness in them. There did seem to be some evidence (at least on the surface) that there may be more of a connection between diet and disease than most people -- myself included – ever considered.

At the very least, this magazine offered some interesting ideas to consider. I couldn't help but think to myself how great it would be if there was some degree of genuineness within its pages. How wonderful it would be if tens of thousands of individuals now sick with terrible diseases could get well ... simply by changing from their present diet to one that consisted primarily of raw "living" foods! As you read further, ask yourself:

... *What are you supposed to eat?*

... *Can a diet change allow your body's immune system to bring healing from serious disease?*

Can This Stuff Be True?

I'm enough of a realist to know that wishful thinking doesn't make for truthful thinking. I often find myself telling others, no matter what the topic or issue, that just because we "want" something to be true doesn't automatically "make" it true.

13

Truth is something that is relevant. If it's not true, then why believe it? If it's not true, then why practice it? If it's not true, then why should we seek to live it or implement it within the fabric of our lives?

In the months that followed, I started reading more along these lines. I found the basic idea about food and its significant influence upon health was very much rooted in modern science. I'd also find a story or two about how average people experienced dramatic healing in their bodies from virtually every chronic disease you can imagine.

Could there be something to these stories? Could this message be true? I wondered. Many of the stories were fascinating. They were also encouraging because they offered hope.

This book summarizes what I first read over a decade ago. My on-again/off-again interest in this topic eventually led me to write about it. After seeing a number of people I personally know get sick, suffer and painfully die this past year I finally decided to write a little bit about nutrition -- and its impact upon human health.

I came to believe those stories I'd read were true largely because I've now personally spoken to many individuals who've experienced what can only be called amazing physical healing through diet change. These are people who went from eating "dead" foods to eating "raw living foods."

For some, extraordinary health benefits came within mere days. For others, healing took place over a period of several weeks or months. The basic diet philosophy and implementation were very similar though.

I have no idea whether the information or personal testimonials inside the pages of this book will affect your thinking in the same way it has affected mine. If so, then you will no doubt find that sense of hope I felt after first reading material like this over a decade ago.

2

An Interview with Larry Jones
Testimony of Healing from Prostate Cancer

A teacher for 37 years, I spent the last 30 of my career at a university here in Missouri. I retired from teaching in 1999 and enjoy living on our family farm in the rolling hills of the north end of the state.

I have always been an active person here on the farm, never been incapacitated in any way, always getting out and working; however, I began to notice that I would tire pretty quickly.

In September of 2005 I was diagnosed with prostate cancer. I had not been feeling well, so my wife suggested that it would be good for me to go and get fully checked out -- including a PSA because of my age, which was 64 at the time. Biopsies showed that I had a very aggressive form of prostate cancer.

I experienced what is probably a normal emotional reaction to this news -- a form of shock. I started thinking that I might not see another Christmas and began to dwell on what was going to happen to my wife Donna, our son Joshua, our daughter Rachel, and her husband Robert after I was gone.

Basically, I started having many thoughts about death. Because I know I would be going home to be with Jesus if I were to die, that part was settled and actually to be looked forward to. However, nobody wants to suffer physically before leaving this world. In addition, nobody wants loved ones to become part of the physical suffering. That thinking process may have been responsible for my realizing that every pain in my body seemed to be magnified. With each pain, whether it was a pulled muscle or a headache, the thought would come to my mind, "*Uh oh, I must have cancer there.*"

After diagnosing me with cancer, the oncologist told me to go home and think about what I wanted to do regarding treatment. Before Donna and I left his office, she asked him how long the surgery, radiation, and chemo would take. She verbalized her guess when she asked him, "*Will it mean at least 2 years of hell?*" He responded that it would.

Donna and I were very depressed for 3 days. Joshua challenged us at the end of those 3 days, saying, "*You both act like you're just giving up! Aren't you going to fight this?*" My thinking was that the best way to fight was to take time to look into what the best place would be to have the traditional treatments done, so I did not respond to the oncologist as quickly as he directed. The man contacted me and said I needed to accept the fact that I had cancer and that if I did not act soon on this, I would die. Again, the only choices in my case were all three -- surgery, radiation, and chemo. He did not, of course, tell me the success rates for those forms of treatment; to find out that they are largely ineffective, my wife had to spend many hours researching.

We came close to choosing to have the surgery done at a very well known hospital. A gentleman was living temporarily in a mobile home on our property, and he had a wealthy uncle who had recently had his prostate removed by a highly respected doctor. When all the connections were set up for me to meet with that doctor, my first reaction was it might be an answer to prayer.

Donna, however, did not have peace about it and was continuing to research. She learned that most men who have had the prostate removed because of cancer have a recurrence of cancer in another part of the body within 10 to 15 years. Both of us agreed that if I endured "2 years of hell" by going through surgery, radiation, and chemo, doing so would not have "cured the cancer" if it would likely return in 10 years or more.

A Nutritional Approach

At that point we were ready to investigate the "Hallelujah Lifestyle" to see if there would be evidence that cancer can be eliminated or controlled through this choice. The cornerstone of this lifestyle is a primarily raw foods diet known as the "Hallelujah Diet."

This diet was first presented to us by Jerri, a lady at our church. After praying, reading books and testimonies, and watching videos about the nutritional approach to healing and health, we decided to reject the traditional route most people take when diagnosed with cancer.

Changing my diet was a major change for both of us. From the very beginning, Donna embraced the changes for herself, but the main reason she did so was in order to help me to live. We gave up foods we were used to eating: all meats, dairy products, white sugar, white flour, and salt (sodium chlorhydrate). But we replaced that diet with the kind of "fuel" that would build our immune systems: raw fruits and veggies, whole grains, nuts, and seeds. That made up about 85 percent of what we ate; the other 15 percent included cooked veggies, soups, stews, and anything that would not harm our bodies. My choosing to drink 64 ounces of carrot juice daily, along with another 64 ounces of water, kept Donna busy as she set timers to remind us both to fit in 2 large salads, juice, and water throughout the day.

Pressures

The medical profession said I should have surgery, chemo, and radiation, which is the route cancer patients have been told to take for decades now. Most people have great faith in doctors and believe the doctors must be right; however, doctors have had very little teaching on the subject of general nutrition and the effect of nutritional excellence on the body.

The idea of treating disease with a nutritional approach is foreign to the average person. News people report about famous people, like Michael Landon and Steve McQueen, who tried to alter their diets when they got sick, hoping that would save their lives. Their deaths were reported without the full story as to what they were actually doing in each stage of their illness. We are left to wonder how close to death they were when they tried the nontraditional approach. We wonder how faithful they were to it. Those facts would help the average person come to a valid conclusion, but the facts are not available to the general public. The end result in the minds of the general public? There are doubts about the validity of nontraditional treatments, including the use of nutrition.

Because most people have been trained to go to a traditional doctor when a health problem arises--and do whatever the doctor prescribes--some people became agitated when they learned that I chose not to follow the doctor's advice. Perhaps they considered it their duty to save me from the certainty of death. I had an aunt who would tell me I should get to the doctor's office, get an operation, undergo the tests, get treatments, and do something to get rid of the cancer. Other reactions to my nontraditional choice have included, "*You're making the wrong choice, and you won't get well*," and "*You should know better,*" and (from a woman who works with our son) "*Your dad's going to*

18

die anyway, so he should get some kind of experimental treatment so they can learn something from his death."

I am a deacon in our church, and my pastor even counseled me against it. He had found some comments on the Internet that were very much against this type of diet, so that influenced his thinking, causing him to conclude that it was the wrong way for me to go.

With all of those negative words of encouragement, I was tempted to question my decision about the Hallelujah Lifestyle. Now and then I would think to myself, "*Have I gone off the deep end?*" As I became more and more informed, those negative thoughts were short lived.

I thank the Lord for my supportive wife. Donna was very much in favor of doing what I wanted to do. Our son, Joshua (then 28 years old), has changed his mind on the subject, but he initially believed that "fighting cancer" meant going the traditional route. He tried hard to tolerate my decision, but he believed my health would be deteriorating quickly. Our daughter, Rachel (then 27), knew very little about the nutritional approach. However, she had worked in a general practitioner's office and saw people come in after surgery and radiation or chemo. They were in such horrible condition that Rachel had decided that if she ever had cancer, she would choose to die before authorizing radiation or chemo. Because Rachel never shared what took place in the doctor's office, we had not been told about her observations--or her decision to never go the traditional route. She was relieved that her mom and dad had come to the same conclusion through studying all options.

No Time or Money on Conventional Medical Treatment

Lorraine Day, M.D., had Stage 4 breast cancer. Dr. Day taught at Loma Linda University in California, and she knew what radiation and chemo would do to her and refused to allow her fellow doctors to use either one on her. Instead, she used a nutritional approach to get well and is a healthy woman today. Chemotherapy destroys the body's immune system. In my opinion, within 20 years or so, somebody will officially determine that chemotherapy has been one of the most barbaric treatments known to man.

I spent no time or money on conventional medical treatment for this prostate cancer, except for diagnosis costs for the biopsies. Our money has been invested instead in books, videos, and training as health ministers so we could help other people. In the summer of 2006, Donna and I went to Shelby, North Carolina, and attended a 4-day retreat at Hallelujah Acres. While there, we heard 128 people share about how they had been healed of everything from cancer to fibromyalgia; heart trouble to diabetes; and arthritis to multiple sclerosis.

The money we did not spend on traditional treatments has instead purchased carrots, Romaine lettuce, spinach, celery, radishes, cucumbers, bok choy, red onions, green onions, zucchini, turnips, mushrooms, peas, broccoli, cauliflower, peppers, asparagus, tomatoes, sweet potatoes, lentils, nuts, beans, flax seeds, whole wheat pasta, sea salt, rice milk, blueberries, peaches, apples, oranges, grapes, raisins, cantaloupes, watermelon, sprouts, a countertop distiller, exercise equipment, BarleyMax, digestive enzymes, and probiotics. We changed our diet all at once -- cold turkey -- on October 15, 2005.

Before and After

Admittedly, I would never have gone on this diet unless it had been for the cancer diagnosis. Soon after making the diet change, I thought I would stick with it for as long as it took to get the cancer under control, then I would return to the Standard American Diet (SAD). I sure have changed my mind about that!

Joel Fuhrman, M.D., author of *Eat to Live*, puts it this way: "...it is exceedingly rare for someone to gain all this knowledge and then go back to unhealthy eating again. They are too informed, and too impressed with their health improvements, to go back and gamble away their newfound health. On top of that, my patients have been weaned from their desire for rich, fatty food."

Giving up unhealthy foods was not hard because I immediately began to feel better. Before the Hallelujah Diet, I would wake up tired after taking a 2-hour afternoon nap. I seldom take naps anymore, nor am I tired at 8 or 9 o'clock at night. I also get up in the morning with plenty of energy and think to myself, "*Good morning, God, what am I going to do today?*"

This diet has not only controlled the cancer, but it has also resulted in my no longer having to take blood pressure or cholesterol medications. (At its peak many years ago, my cholesterol level was 685. The triglyceride serum the first time around was too thick to test. That alone should have motivated me to do something more than take meds for the problems; both my mom and dad died of heart disease.)

A year before the cancer diagnosis, I went to a chiropractor because of trouble with my leg bone welding to my hip socket, which made walking very painful. After six treatments, however, I felt much better. Fast-forward one year, and the pain in my hip was returning, just before starting the Hallelujah Diet. Amazingly, I never had to go back to the chiropractor. With the right fuel in my body, the hip pain went away--and so did every other pain in my body for that matter -- and I am now 68 years old.

I feel very healthy. I lost about 40 pounds, and Donna lost about 30. I do not subscribe to a drug plan through Medicare because I do not need to take any medications. Working here on the farm keeps me busy with building and

21

repairing fences, mowing lawns and pastures, and doing general maintenance.

Donna had a low level of lupus for 15 years; during that time it tested positive each year, and she had to stay out of the sun as much as possible, always wearing a heavy-duty sunblock when she was outside. After a short time on the Hallelujah Diet, tests showed that lupus vanished--all symptoms are gone. To God be the glory for healing my wife as she supported me by changing her diet!

Two summers ago, we went to a water park in Kansas City, Missouri. Donna was in the sun with me in 95-degree temperatures, yet she suffered no ill effects whatsoever. Had she still had lupus, she could have been hospitalized for spending hours in the hot sun in the middle of the day in a swimsuit.

Often when I tell people they can get rid of their health problems, they agree that what they are eating may be causing their health problems, but they are not willing to do what is necessary in order to get healthy. Some agree that eating raw (living) foods would be better than eating mostly all cooked (dead) foods, but they want to simply add living foods to the dead foods they are already eating.

Donna likes to explain the futility of eating good foods but not eliminating the bad foods, all the while expecting the body to heal itself, by using this illustration: Picture yourself taking a shower to clean off dirt, but somebody keeps throwing more dirt at you. You will soon realize that you will not make much progress until you stop the dirt coming at you! Until you quit eating the foods that are harming your body, healing will not take place.

I have not been back to the oncologist since the December following the cancer diagnosis in 2005. So I have not received official confirmation that the cancer has gone from my body. The last time I had my PSA level checked it was a bit higher than it was at the time of my diagnosis, but the number did not upset me. However, it did motivate me to continue taking Curcumin, a supplement to combat inflammation and fight free radicals, and to add a Vitamin B17 supplement and foods containing B17 to my diet.

Check It Out

The books and videos below will help you get started in learning about how you can do your part in bringing about a healthy body. Information and testimonies from individuals who have overcome every imaginable disease can be found on the Hallelujah Acres website at www.hacres.com. Individual "*Healing for Life*" DVD's on each of the following can be obtained from the same website: Arthritis & Osteoporosis; Cancer; Diabetes; Fibromyalgia & Lupus; and Weight Issues. "*Healing Cancer from the Inside Out,*" a video by Mike Anderson, is another excellent resource at that website.

Meat... T. Colin Campbell's book, *The China Study* is summarized in The China Project. He reports on a huge study done by American, Chinese, and British researchers who substantiated that as the amount of animal foods increase in the diet, even in relatively small amounts, (and even lean meats and chicken), so did the cancers that are common in our country. Virtually no heart attacks in those Chinese who had a vegetarian diet. Almost no heart attacks in Chinese who had a diet rich in natural plant foods with less than 10 percent of their calories from animal foods.

Water... Previous generations did not have to contend with drinking water that contains chemicals from the runoff produced by modern agricultural methods. My wife and I drink distilled water. We even have filters on our showers to keep chlorine, fluoride, and other chemicals from being absorbed into our bodies.

Sugar... We all know that sugar is very bad for the body, causing the immune system to be unable to function as it should.

Milk Products... Dr. Joel Fuhrman asks, "*Are Dairy Foods Protecting Us from Osteoporosis?*" in his book, Eat to Live. Osteoporosis is a major health problem in our country, in spite of the fact that our country consumes more dairy products than any other place on earth. Dr. Fuhrman explains why "*the only way to prevent osteoporosis and have strong bones is to exercise and to stop the causes of high urinary calcium excretion*" by being on a diet similar to the diet I have been telling you about. If you prefer a video, Dr. Fuhrman has two, "*The Greatest Diet on Earth*" and "*The Greatest Diet on Earth II.*"

Exercise... God's Way to Ultimate Health by George Malkmus recommends a simple, inexpensive exercise program. This book also shares many testimonies, along with pictures and names, of people who had wonderful results after being on the Hallelujah Diet.

Sunshine, Fresh Air, and Sleep... These are very important, too, and are discussed in most books and videos.

Chemicals in both foods and the environment affect health. Chronic diseases are increasing. I encourage skeptics to find out why. Take a look at videos by Dr. Lorraine Day, especially "*Diseases Don't Just Happen,*" "*Cancer Doesn't Scare Me Anymore,*" and "*You Can't Improve on God!*"

Imagine how wonderful life could be if you could get rid of your health problems! God gave us marvelous, self-healing bodies; let's do whatever we must do to see that healing take place. My e-mail address is *rjones@nemr.net.*

24

3
An Interview with
Justin Gingerella
Testimony of Healing from Throat Cancer

I am a musician. I live in southern California right now, but I used to live in Seattle, Washington.

I'd been living in Seattle for a while, working as a web designer within the high-tech industry for corporations such as Microsoft, Amazon.com and Starbucks. I also worked as the art director for a company called FreerInternet.com. I did web design work full-time for years and performed music on the side.

When I was working in the corporate world I didn't have a clear vision of what I wanted to do with music, even though I knew deep down inside that it's what I wanted to do with my life. I'd played drums until I was about 23 years old, before working in the tech industry. But I'd always wanted to sing, write songs and play guitar.

I was doing well both professionally and financially at the time, at least by the standards most people use to gauge those things. They were great experiences. But things changed one day when I was working at Microsoft and went to the doctor's office for a routine checkup.

"The Cancer Had Already Spread"

When I went in for my checkup that day, the doctor pressed his hands to my throat to examine it and he felt something there that didn't feel right. So he began a process to find out what was going on.

He'd felt some lumps in my throat and wanted me to get an ultrasound. I made an appointment and had one done. It revealed the presence of some nodules in my throat. Since those can be either benign or active, the doctors then performed a needle aspiration to check them out further. Things were still inconclusive after that. The doctors then wanted to perform a surgery and take a piece of my thyroid gland out. So that's what I decided to let them do.

At this point, I'd been singing for a period of time. I'd even put out my first EP. Having surgery performed on my throat was scary. The doctor told me surgeries in this area could result in me losing my voice permanently.

I was obviously very concerned about it. I really wanted to perform as a musician and I was just beginning to get back heavily into it.

A couple weeks after the doctors took out part of my thyroid they told me I definitely had thyroid cancer. They were going to have to go back into the same area and cut the rest of the thyroid out to try and remove all the cancer cells.

The doctors went back in during another surgery and removed the rest of my thyroid. That meant I'd now gone through surgery in the same spot twice.

When I was recovering from that second surgery the doctors set up an appointment for me to have another scan in order to see if all the cancer was removed. As it turned out, the cancer had already spread out of the thyroid area and was heading down into the area of my lung. At this point, things were looking pretty bad. When I was 19 yrs old I had to have a lung removed, so I only had one lung now.

The doctors were very concerned the cancer had spread out of the area of the thyroid. They also expressed concern

26

about how fast it was spreading. They were headed towards doing some chemo, among other things.

I was obviously very scared about all of this. I was really thinking hard about these procedures.

"Get Out of that Hospital Right Now"

Just after going back into the hospital to get my first sessions of some radiation treatment, I received a phone call from a man named Jerrod Sessler. Jerrod was one of my web clients. One of my businesses at the time involved doing some web design work for Jerrod.

Jerrod was a Nascar race driver and had his own website. He was contacting me to do some site update work. When he called me at the hospital I said, "*I can't Jerrod. I'm in kind of a bad situation right now.*" He asked me what was going on, so I told him.

The doctors had just begun treating me with a small radiation pill. Jerrod said, "*You need to get out of that hospital right now. You need to get to my class on Wednesday night. I'm going to show you how to beat cancer.*" When Jerrod explained a little bit more about this option, it seemed like something that was right for me at that moment … better than going the way of poisonous chemo.

Hearing I had cancer, for me, was sort of like experiencing phases of thoughts and emotions. Most people are aware of the stages of grief individuals can go through. For me, there was first disbelief about the cancer diagnosis. Then there was a little bit of, "*Why me?*" Then there was some anger.

But then a determination came to me. You can choose to feel sorry for yourself and go into a dark place. Or you can choose to take on an attitude that says, "*I'm going to beat this thing and I'm going to attack it with everything possible.*"

For me, the amount of clarity I received after hearing this diagnosis … about my life and what I wanted to do

27

with it ... what I wanted to accomplish in relation to what I've done so far ... all came into focus. This included where I lived, the people I'd loved or hurt. It all came into play the first night I laid my head on the pillow on that first night after receiving that diagnosis.

Facing the idea that you could be experiencing your own mortality soon can bring clarity to your thinking. It can remove the fog that comes with just floating through life. If I had to say there was a "blessing" part of a double-edged sword then that's what it was for me. I finally realized what I wanted to do with my life. I knew the things I needed to change. I realized the things I wanted to focus on more. That difficult time was a place where I personally began "real living."

I had what I thought was a pretty amazing life prior to this ... as far as things I've done and places I've been. But the funny thing about this was it all felt like a dream after the diagnosis. It felt like everything had just flashed by so quickly. I think this may be because I was always "looking for the next big thing" or "wishing for that." Until you get this clarity of thinking you can't enjoy the moments of your life as you're in them. But now there was clarity for me.

"Things Started Changing Immediately"

When Jerrod told me to leave the hospital I was open to listening to what he had to say. The clarity about how I wanted my life to go at that point allowed me to be more open to the information he began sharing with me about changing my diet. Before that point, I probably wouldn't have been as open to the idea. I'd have probably called Jerrod a nutcase. But this was something that I was now willing to consider.

I went to Jerrod's first class, and to be honest, I was a little skeptical. But I brought the girl who was my girlfriend at the time with me to the class as well. We listened to everything. We saw some videos. Not only did I see others' testimonies of healing, but also the food science taken into account with this nutritional approach to what we should and shouldn't be eating. I really saw how so much of the food consumed today is processed in a way that is purely for profit even though it's unhealthy.

To this day, I think that if the cancer ever came back (or if I knew anyone who got sick with cancer) it just makes total sense to me that being fully healthy is about living with your body in the cleanest state possible. That just makes sense, even if the decision is made to fight the cancer using conventional medical treatments.

What did I have to lose? It was really a mind over matter thing. I went home and literally threw away every single thing in my cupboards. Then I went to the store the next day and started eating mostly raw.

I also started juicing carrot juice and wheatgrass. To me, I really believe that was really important. I've seen other testimonies involving people who didn't follow the prescribed raw diet that I followed but they overcame serious health conditions by juicing. I've seen videos of individuals who overcame their problems with just carrot juice and wheatgrass. That was years after I began this juicing combination, but their testimonies really blew me away.

I changed to the mostly raw diet "cold turkey." I juiced every day and ate raw every day. I consumed about 85-90% raw food, and the cooked portion consisted of meals such as wheat pasta with sauce or organic vegetable soups … things like that. Most of the time, however, it was raw fruits, nuts, and giant salads.

Things started changing immediately. The first thing I noticed was how other physical problems I'd dealt with for years went away. There were things I thought I'd have for the rest of my life because they were just a part of being who I am.

There were stomach problems. I regularly had trouble sleeping at night. And I'd also been having headaches when I went to bed.

All of my stomach problems simply went away. I didn't have one problem after I began eating raw. The headaches ... the thumping in my head at night when I put my head against the pillow ... it was completely gone. I also slept like a baby. That's when I knew eating this way was already a better way to go.

In addition, I was about 20 pounds heavier than before starting the raw diet. My skin started looking different too. About 6 weeks after changing to a raw diet I didn't look the same; my skin didn't look the same. I almost looked like I did when I was 18.

"The Doctors Were Completely Baffled"

I was on this mostly raw diet for just over a year, adhered to it strictly, and then went back to the doctor's to have another scan done of my throat and chest areas. I wanted to see how things were progressing.

To be honest, I had major anxiety over this scan. Waiting for the results was obviously the hardest part.

When the new scans were completed the doctors were completely baffled. They put my new scans up against the prior ones. There wasn't even one trace of cancer!

Compared to the prior scan I had a year before, the new pictures were completely clean. When they told me the results I was stunned.

At first, even the doctors thought their machine was broken. They called USC Medical Center to speak with some technicians about these test results. But as it turned out, there really was nothing there. That was it for me.

That was 6 years ago. And I've never been back to the doctors there for any more treatment. My only trips to the doctor's office since then have been to get regular blood tests for the thyroid medication I need to take because I no longer have a thyroid gland.

I now have a reference point, a confidence builder, for fighting off cancer. That's the way I look at it anyway.

When I was cured from cancer my diet was very "vegan," with an abundance of raw foods. I've modified it a little bit now and would call my current diet "vegetarian." It seems to work well for me at the moment. But I want to get back to my original raw food diet as much as possible.

When I first changed my diet it was actually kind of fun. The hardest part about maintaining the diet for me has been slipping back into "convenience" and the niche foods associated with my particular demographic area.

When I initially changed to a raw diet, my girlfriend at the time changed her diet with me. I think I'll be indebted to her forever because she encouraged me to stay on track every day. She was always ready to try a new recipe and learn how to prepare foods in a new way. She helped make it fun.

Most people think, "*A diet of mostly raw foods will limit me.*" But the reality is that those people are limited. I can almost guarantee that they are the ones who always go to the same 3 or 4 restaurants, and they're the ones who eat about the same 10 things all the time ... and they've probably been on that same track for the last 10 years. They think they're freer because they can eat anything they want. The thing is, they always end up in the same zone.

The raw food diet forced me to try all new foods, while discovering amazing new ways to prepare it. I experienced new tastes that I'd never experienced before in my life. Then I began to see how new versions of things could be created. Mealtime got really creative and fun. This meant I ended up with more variety and an ability to try things I probably never would have tried before.

The recipes out nowadays for raw foods include everything under the sun, including things like tacos, ice creams, brownies and peach tarts. Everything you've eaten in the past has a raw food variant to it ... in addition to a million other things you've never experienced before.

The thing is, you have to be willing to put in a certain amount of time and effort to discover them. Most people aren't, which is why they're not more open to the idea of changing their diet to a healthy one; that's the reality of it. But facing something like cancer will definitely give you a motivation to try something new.

There is a process I now go through to try and live in all of the moments of my life. My life has slowed down and it gives me more joy. I think so many people's lives are "sped up" because they're never "in the moment." So then life just flies past them and they never really experience anything. It's like being in sleep mode on autopilot.

After being diagnosed with something like cancer, if you're open to it, the awareness and self-actualization process can really give you a second chance at life. You can really start living the way you should have been living the whole time. That's how I feel about it anyway.

With a new lease on life, I knew I was going to be doing music. I was going to go into it full-bore, with all of my heart, and have a lot to say with positive music.

It was joy and therapy for me to begin making music. I made a decision to get rid of things in my life that were financially paying me well but not feeding my soul in any way, shape or form. Sitting in a cubicle was not the way I was going to end my life.

So I quit Microsoft and I quit every job I had and went full-bore into music. I started my own companies and began to personally align my life with the dreams I had -- which is what I should've been doing the whole time anyway.

"Be Willing to Try This"

As far as I know, the status of my health right now is excellent. If I hadn't seen this diet work for other people then I would have been skeptical about it with regards to my own recovery. But Jerrod himself was living proof, and others he has helped were living proof that it can work.

There are a ton of others you can find out there who have stories just like mine. What would a skeptic say to that? What are you going to say to somebody who has changed to a raw food diet and beaten diabetes or cancer without seeing a doctor? Most people don't make this stuff up.

When you educate yourself about the "science of food" it should really hit home. Human beings cook their food, killing all the natural nutrients that keep them healthy. We're also the only creatures that drink another creature's milk. Those were the first 2 things that hit me like a ton of bricks and made me think we might be on the wrong path with regards to the Standard American Diet.

In addition to these things, it's not hard to understand that if a company can make a bunch of money by adding artificial ingredients to a product then they'll do it most of the time. The health problems of this country have skyrocketed since the advent of modern, mass food production. There's no other correlation to come up with other than what we're eating.

I would challenge anyone who is considering a diet like this to find the negatives. What are the negatives to being healthier? It's not like eating high-quality foods is some sort of voodoo that we don't know is good or not. It's not like that. Everyone knows eating healthier can produce positive health results. It's just about whether or not you really want it. If you want health then you'll be willing to try this. If not, then you won't.

It was the same way with my music. For the last 5 years I've put out 4 records, toured the entire United States and had amazing experiences that most people will never have. The best part has been getting to meet new people who've connected with my music on a personal level. They email me or come up to me and thank me ... and none of this would have happened if I'd stayed in that cubicle. And if I'd never been diagnosed with cancer then I would've never got that clarity of vision about where I wanted my life to go. I really got the boost behind me to *"just do it."*

I invite readers to visit my website at justinblack.net for free music downloads. There'll be free songs available if you're interested.

. . . .

Justin Gingerella's website, which contains videos of Justin playing, along with free music downloads, can be found at: **www.JustinBlack.net**

4
What Does the Science Say?

Before discussing what scientific studies teach about diet and its effect upon health, allow me to quickly mention one important issue that sets the stage for everything discussed in this chapter. It has to do with the fact we're all very biased!

Our biases are particularly strong when it comes to things we like and dislike. None of us are impartial or without preferences. And I'm talking here about more than whether we like certain kinds of food or not; I'm speaking about the beliefs we currently associate with food.

The reality of the existence of such biases means scientific facts never simply "speak objectively" because they're interpreted subjectively by each individual. While objective truth does exist, how we choose to interpret data depends upon many things, especially our biases and current beliefs. This is why different people often look upon the same data, yet come to very different interpretations and conclusions about what the data "says."

Western medicine is truly a marvel when it comes to certain things. For example, one place it really excels is in the area of trauma. When it comes to treating certain injuries that have occurred due to accidents some of the results are often nothing short of amazing.

How many of us have seen stories on television involving incredible surgeries that restore health from accidental injury? Such human dramas are perfect examples of how we can appreciate the excellent training doctors receive along certain lines and what a blessing Western medicine can be.

There is another side of things, however. Western medicine's track record for treating chronic illness and disease isn't very good at all. Exactly why this is the case is open for debate. There is abundant scientific evidence that shows diet may dramatically impact health ... both positively and negatively.

In spite of this research, however, many doctors seem to be in the dark (and sometimes hostile) to the notion that many illnesses are diet related. They are also often skeptical of any suggestion that changing the foods one eats can often enable a body to heal itself of diseases labeled as "incurable" from a medical standpoint.

The point here is that even though all doctors are trained to treat disease scientifically, there seems to be gaps in both knowledge and consensus among physicians about what science has "revealed" concerning the connection between diet and disease. You need to be aware of this.

There are probably a number of reasons why some physicians are open to the idea that nutrition can dramatically impact health, while others are not. But I'm sure the fact that human nature is biased (and this includes the human nature possessed by medical doctors and researchers) is one of those reasons. There are many reasons, identifiable or not, that we believe some things but not others.

Another reality we have to wrestle with is the fact many people simply choose to believe whatever they WANT to believe is true ... instead of being open to having their views changed. In other words, many people are attracted to opinions and analysis that apparently confirm what they already believe (or want to be true) instead of being open to having their views challenged in any way.

Changing views and opinions means re-thinking and re-evaluating what one already thinks is true about the world and their place in it. That may be a rather unpleasant experience. So it's often much easier to simply hold fast to what one already thinks is true or wants to be true.

In light of this, what do I think the science "says" about diet and healing? In my opinion, the evidence overwhelmingly points to the fact that poor diet is often a leading cause of disease. In addition, a healthy diet can offer many disease sufferers (and those who want to maintain health) the ingredients their bodies need to often heal themselves.

We will only scratch the surface of a discussion about evidence here. It's much easier to link to references and additional information resources at **LivingFoodCures.com** for this purpose. So please use this site as a future reference for more supporting data.

A Remarkable Statement

Consider the following passage from chapter 7 of Dr. Joel Fuhrman's book, "*Eat To Live*," one of the most remarkable books on the subject of diet and health in this generation:

> We are living among an addicted population of compulsive eaters, creating allergic and sickly individuals. Eat and live like most Americans and you will eventually suffer an assortment of ailments, like most Americans.
>
> Good health is not merely the absence of disease. Good health assumes protection from disease in the future and can be predicted only by a healthy lifestyle and diet.
>
> You cannot buy your health; you must earn it through healthy living. Visiting physicians, acupuncturists, chiropractors, homeopaths, naturopaths, osteopaths, and other health providers cannot make you

healthy. You can receive symptomatic relief for you condition, but treatments do not make you healthy.

For most people, illness means putting their fate in the hands of doctors and complying with their recommendations - recommendations that typically involve taking drugs for the rest of their lives while they watch their health gradually deteriorate. People are completely unaware that most illnesses are self-induced and can be reversed with aggressive nutritional methods.

Both patients and physicians act as though everyone's medical problems are generic, or assumed to be the normal consequence of aging. They believe that chronic illness is just what we all must expect. Unfortunately, the medical-pharmaceutical business has encouraged people to believe that health problems are hereditary and that we need to swallow poisons to defeat our genes. This is almost always untrue. We all have genetic weaknesses, but those weaknesses never get a chance to express themselves until we abuse our body with many, many years of mistreatment. Never forget, 99 percent of your genes are programmed to keep you healthy. The problem is that we never let them do their job.

My clinical experience over the past ten years has shown me that almost all the major illnesses that plague Americans are reversible with aggressive nutritional changes designed to undo the damage caused by years of a eating disease-causing diet. The so-called balanced diet that most Americans eat is causing the diseases Americans get.

These conditions, and many others, can be effectively prevented or treated through superior nutrition. As their medical problems gradually melt away, patients can be slowly weaned off the medications they have been prescribed.

Food Is the Cure

Patients are told that food has nothing to do with the diseases they develop. Dermatologists insist that food has nothing to do with acne, rheumatologists insist that food has nothing to do with rheumatoid arthritis, and gastroenterologists insist that food has nothing to do with irritable and inflammatory bowel disease. Even cardiologists have been resistant to accept the accumulating evidence that arteriosclerosis is entirely avoidable. Most of them still believe that coronary artery disease and angina require the invasive treatment of surgery and are not reversible with nutritional intervention. Most physicians have no experience in treating disease naturally with nutritional excellence, and some physicians who don't know about it are convinced it is not possible.

Not only are common disorders such as asthma associated with increased body weight and our disease-causing diet, but in my experience these diseases are also curable with superior nutrition in the majority of cases. Asthma is an example of a disease considered irreversible that I watch resolve regularly.

My patients routinely make complete and predictable recovery from these illnesses, predominantly through aggressive dietary changes. I am always delighted to meet new patients who are ready to take responsibility for their own health and well-being.

You can watch a new you being made by the wisdom of your body, and this new you will result in all your systems and organs, including your brain, functioning better. Depression, fatigue, anxiety, and allergies are also related to our improper diet. The brain and immune system are able to withstand stress better when our body is properly nourished.

I am neither a research scientist nor a writer by profession. I am a practicing physician who sees at least five thousand patients a year. I work with these patients, educating them and motivating them to do more than others have asked them to do. The results I see with my patients are thrilling. Diseases that are considered irreversible I see reversed on a daily basis.

The overwhelming majority of my patients with high blood pressure are able to normalize their readings and eventually go off their medication. The majority of my patients with angina can end their symptoms of coronary artery disease in the first few months on the diet I prescribe. Most of the rest make recovery, but it takes longer. The point is, they do recover.

More than 90 percent of my Type II diabetics are able to eventually discontinue their insulin within the first month. More than 80 percent of my chronic headache and migraine sufferers recover without medication, after years of looking for relief with various physicians, including headache specialists.

Some people, especially other physicians, may be skeptical. There are so many exaggerated and false claims made in the health field, especially by those selling so-called natural remedies. Nevertheless, it is wrong to underestimate the results obtainable through appropriate but rigorous nutritional intervention. Even many of my patients with autoimmune illnesses (such as lupus, rheumatoid arthritis, asthma, and hyperthyroidism) are able to recover and throw away their medications. The results are so spectacular that I am subjected to skepticism and even periodic expressions of anger from other physicians.[3]

Aren't Dr Fuhrman's comments remarkable? Here is a man who helps thousands of patients experience dramatic bodily healing every year using nutrition -- in harmony with conventional medicine. Yet many of his colleagues don't want to hear about it.

Isn't there a certain element of "proof" in testimonials? Isn't there enough data up to this point in order to justify extensive testing of nutritional approaches to wellness based upon the success of physicians like Dr Fuhrman, and many others, who also see breakthroughs in their patients' health? Of course there is. But in the words of Christ, some information is only meaningful to "those who have ears to hear."

What Causes Many Diseases?

According to the American Cancer Society's document, "Cancer Facts & Figures 2009," there will be an estimated 562,340 cancer deaths and 1,479,350 new cancer cases in the U.S. alone.[4] Cancer is the second leading disease causing death in this country -- second only to heart disease. Yet throughout many parts of Asia, cancer is rare, especially digestive related ones like colon cancer.

While there may be any number of causes for cancer, there is a huge amount of scientific evidence indicating cancer is a disease that often occurs because of the failure of a body's immune system. And the immune system is dramatically affected by what a person eats.

How many times have you heard of somebody having a cancerous tumor removed from his or her body ... only to have it recur again within a short period of time? Why did that happen? Because the root cause of the disease apparently wasn't dealt with.

A number of factors could play into a failure of an individual's immune system. There could be something in the environment. A number of researched articles argue that chemicals used in public water treatment facilities may cause certain illnesses. But if that's true then it makes sense a person's diet could play an even bigger role. Diet may be the most significant factor in determining whether or not an immune system functions properly.

A healthy immune system is one that "handles" cells that tend to become cancerous. Every person has a small amount of cancer cells in their body at any given moment. A healthy immune system, however, is able to handle those cancer cells and keep them from becoming tumors inside the body. Dr. Rowen Pfeifer explains:

"When you have a healthy person on a good diet, you see a lot of white blood cells - they're very active - moving around. It reminds me of the old Pacman game because they're gobbling up the mutated cells. You can actually see those cells engulfing things that don't belong in your body, getting rid of them, and then moving on. However, with patients on a diet high in sugar and white flour, you see only a few white blood cells and they are dormant - just lying there, drugged and unable to do their job ... So now you get these mutated cells that become pre-cancerous and cancerous. As more of them accumulate they begin bunching together ... In other words, you have a tumor or cancer developing."[5]

While other factors may be involved, the most obvious common denominator to many forms of cancer is food. When individuals move to the West from parts of the world where cancer is rare, and then adapt Western eating habits, they begin acquiring cancer at the same rate as other Westerners.

Studies comparing raw plant-based diets against animal based ones continuously show that animal food is harmful to human health. Animal food products consumed in large enough amounts may actually be toxic over a period of time. Some scientific findings even indicate that certain types of cancer, such as prostrate cancer, are dramatically impacted by diet.[6]

One of the most significant books ever written about the relationship between diet and disease is Dr. T. Colin Campbell's work entitled, *"The China Study."*[7] Its subtitle reads, *"The Most Comprehensive Study of Nutrition Ever Conducted and the Startling Implications for Diet, Weight Loss and Long-term Health."*

Years ago, Dr. Campbell worked with malnourished children in the Philippines. He tried to find out why so many Filipino children were diagnosed with liver cancer. He noted that the primary goal of the nutrition project he worked on was to make sure these children were getting as much protein as possible.

Dr. Campbell discovered that the children who consumed the highest amounts of protein in their diets were the ones likeliest to get liver cancer. So he began collecting reports from around the world to see if there were any similarities. That eventually led him to further study nutrition and its connection with disease.

In what became a 20-year study, Dr. Campbell worked in partnership with Oxford and Cornell universities and the Chinese Academy of Preventive Medicine. The result was groundbreaking research that evidenced more than 8000 associations between diet and disease.

Dr. Campbell concluded that individuals who consume the most "animal-based" diets get the most chronic diseases. And those who eat more "plant-based" diets tend to avoid chronic diseases.

To be fair, it must be acknowledged that there are many scientists who would disagree with Dr. Campbell's conclusions. And while his work may be said to be "comprehensive," the scientific community as a whole would not regard it as "conclusive."

The fact remains, however, that his body of research is extremely comprehensive in scope. It demonstrates clear scientific evidence in favor of a plant-based diet and why those who want to defeat or avoid disease should consider embracing veganism ... while simultaneously avoiding all animal-based food products.

The data also seems to hold true over a whole range of prominent chronic illnesses afflicting most people in the West. Whether the subject is heart disease or various types of cancer, it seems as if diet can play a major role in either hurt or healing.

Dr. Joel Fuhrman who is both a medical doctor and nutritional counselor, noted, "... *recent data from Harvard University has shown that when women's diets are low in animal fats, or if they leave it out completely, breast cancer is less likely to occur. For men, diet changes seem to matter just as much. Here, we're seeing particular benefits not only from avoiding meat, but also from avoiding dairy products. A substantial amount of evidence shows that avoiding dairy can reduce the risk of prostate cancers by a very substantial degree.*"[8]

The False Logic in Many Food Studies

Have you heard that you should be on a low-fat diet because dietary fats are the big health problem today? Or have you heard that fish oil, which contains omega-3 fatty acids, helps prevent heart disease? Probably.

Such ideas are now widespread thanks to a number of research studies that have been well publicized by the media over the years. The problem with many food studies in relation to health, however, is their results end up making wrong comparisons.

For example, diet studies comparing "low fat" foods against "high-fat" foods of similar quality are certainly going to appear to be healthier. And studies touting benefits of omega-3 fats within fish, while ignoring the increased health risks from fish toxicity (not to mention the fact that omega-

3 fat from plants is healthier), leave readers with false impressions.

Comparing 2 different kinds of processed or animal-based foods against each other in order to make the case that the slightly better choice is actually "healthy" is false logic. Just because one food product seems to be healthier for human beings compared to another food product in a certain study doesn't mean it's good for human beings to consume overall.

Imagine if a health study came out saying it's "healthier" for human lungs to inhale only 3 packs of cigarette smoke a day instead of 4 packs. Would that mean smoking 3 packs of cigarettes is healthy? Of course not! But that is exactly how the media does comparison reporting on the results of many food research studies.

The fact is, when the whole varieties of data comparing processed or animal-based food products against plant-based vegetables and fruits (for nutritional quality and health benefits) are scrutinized, plant-based foods win by a landslide. The results aren't even close.

As far back as 1996 a report came out stating there were 337 studies by the National Cancer Institute that correlated longevity and health in humans with consumption of fruits and vegetables. The report stated:

1. Vegetables and fruits protect against all types of cancers if consumed in large enough quantities. Hundreds of scientific studies document this. The most prevalent cancers in our country are mostly plant-food-deficiency diseases.

2. Raw vegetables have the most powerful anti-cancer properties of all foods.

3. Studies on the cancer-reducing effects of vitamin pills containing various nutrients (such as folate, vitamin

C and E) get mixed reviews; sometimes they show slight benefit, but most show no benefit. Occasionally studies show that taking isolated nutrients is harmful, as was discussed earlier regarding beta-carotene.

4. Beans, in general, not just soy, have additional anti-cancer benefits against reproductive cancers, such as breast and prostate cancer[9]

Nutrition supplement manufacturers make millions of dollars each year selling pills that promise to supply what bodies need to stay healthy. Many people choose that option because they think they can take a few vitamins and supplements and then eat anything they want and still remain free of disease. Unfortunately, life doesn't work that way ... at least not yet. The key to health and weight loss is eating vegetables, fruits, beans and nuts, plus other raw and whole foods -- with vegetables at the top of the list.

Diet and Longevity

Many studies conducted over the years show vegetarians live longer than non-vegetarians do.[10] But what's interesting is that these studies seem to indicate that even if someone isn't 100% vegetarian they'll generally be healthier if they consume large amounts of raw vegetables and fruits than those who claim to be vegetarians but don't consume large amounts of those living foods. Somebody who claims to be "vegetarian" yet eats lots of processed foods out of a box purchased from a health food store (instead of raw and whole foods) doesn't enjoy significant health benefits. Apparently, health and well being are found within raw living foods as opposed to meats, dairy or even "vegetarian" type processed foods.

Dr. William Castelli writes, "*We tend to scoff at vegetarians, but they're doing much better than we are. Vegans have cholesterol levels so low, they almost never get heart attacks. Their average blood cholesterol is about 125 and we've never seen anyone in the Farmingham study have a heart attack with a level below 150.*[11]

Any adult with an average IQ knows smoking isn't healthy. And most everyone knows smoking is associated with lung cancer. But what is amazing is that rates of lung cancer are as much as 1/5 lower in countries where the population consumes high amounts of vegetables and fruits ... in spite of the fact that smoking is also prevalent. So it appears raw fruits and vegetables offer powerful disease-preventing qualities even in cancer cases directly caused by a bad health habit like smoking.

If you want to avoid health problems such as cancer, heart disease, high-blood pressure and diabetes then you should avoid all meat and dairy products.[12] Shunning unhealthy foods and ingesting the right ones may significantly impact your health. To put things even more simply, the more green salads you consume the greater the odds of you living much longer.[13]

5

An Interview with
Judy Livingstone
Testimony of Healing from Multiple Sclerosis

I live with my husband at home, amid beautiful woods in the state of Maine. I don't refer to myself as "retired," but I don't work outside of the home.

About 21 years ago, I lived in the Florida Keys. I was working as a cashier in a busy supermarket during the winter season, which is very busy down there. As I worked, I began to lose part of my visual sight. Some of the keys on the keyboard were disappearing on me as I was typing. I left work and went to see a medical doctor right away.

My primary care doctor suggested I go see an eye doctor at first. I went to see a specialist at Miami-Dade hospital. While there, I underwent a lot of testing, including a "patch-light" test where they would sort of pop lights on and off and I'd have to identify where the lights were. The doctors eventually decided to run an MRI.

After results came back from the MRI, the medical staff saw 4 lesions on my brain. That's when they determined I had Multiple Sclerosis. Those lesions were indicative of a deterioration of the nylon sheets on the nerve endings of my brain, and this appeared as "white matter" on the MRI.

There are what I call "transmitters," that go from the brain across certain areas of the head, and they were beginning to tell parts of my body to shut down. At that point, there were only 4 affected areas, but they were beginning to affect the visual functions of my eyes.

I'd heard about this disease before but never quite understood it. When I was diagnosed, at 40 years of age, I thought that I was probably just going to end up being a vegetable. I figured it would affect my nerves, muscles and organs, and then eventually, as time went on, it would eventually take me.

Upon leaving his office, the doctor told me to read all I could about this disease. But then he said I should put all the literature away and just live my life. I felt as if he was saying that he wanted me to know about it, but then wanted me to take each experience as it came and not worry about the next symptom. He was suggesting that I enjoy life as I could, in between symptoms, without worrying what was going to happen to me next.

At that point of my diagnosis, the doctor felt the disease was "slow progressive." He felt like it would just slowly get progressively worse. He didn't recommend any medication for me at that point. But he did have me take home a chart that went on my refrigerator.

The doctor wanted me to look at the dots on it so I could square off the areas I could see each time I looked at it. I'd mark this down so the doctor could read this chart on my next visit. That would help him see how things were going. Within a couple of weeks my vision returned.

"I Really Started Feeling Desperate"

With MS, as you get older, your immune system can sort of shut down a bit. Things don't want to work correctly. And later on, when the disease finally became "full-blown," I realized that stress was also a factor with MS.

Up to that point in my life I had never deviated from what is known as the "Standard American Diet." I ate 3 meals a day. I drank coffee. Never did I think that this was

49

some sort of "self-abuse process." It was how I'd been raised. But had I known back then what I know now, I don't think I would have suffered nearly as long with this disease as I did.

I eventually felt really sick from the disease once again. This time, it had to do with my legs. As a result, I had to come back home ... to Maine.

I was beginning to get wobbly and unsteady. It wouldn't happen consistently, but I'd get attacks and certain motor skills were affected. For me, instead of my legs shutting down entirely, I felt as if I couldn't walk straight. And I also felt as if I was going "downhill" all the time.

My legs were starting to feel as if electric shocks were going down them all the time. So I began searching out medications, from both my primary care physician and neurologist, to try and deal with the symptoms I was having.

Those medications didn't help me at all because the more I took, the less mobile I became. The medicine itself affected my mobility. So the meds didn't stop the disease, nor halt its progression.

I was eventually prescribed oxygen to use on a regular basis because I was really getting sick with cluster headaches. When I had those headaches, I had to take in about 8 liters of oxygen and breath it for 12 minutes. It was either do it at home or do it at an emergency room ... which is why we got a tank at home.

I also was given a walker and an AFO lift-brace for one foot because I was beginning to drag it. I started wearing that AFO support on my foot so I could pick it up without tripping on it.

I eventually went to a doctor here in the state of Maine in 2002 and had another MRI done. That scan showed 8 lesions on my brain. So the disease had progressed.

I really started feeling desperate. I would have been willing to go out of the country to get better if I could have. I was willing to go anywhere if I could find a fix for this

50

because I knew I was getting worse as each day went by. I didn't think that I'd even be able to hold my first grandchild in my arms because I didn't know they'd be sturdy enough to hold him.

"You Can Get Better"

I'd been going to a local church here for 11 years. (I was on the worship team). One Sunday, a man came to church. He was blind and had a Seeing-Eye dog. It happened to be on a day that I was singing.

When I got up to sing, I told one of the gentlemen in our church that I couldn't get up and that I was losing my balance. I confided that I needed some help to get down off the stage. He said, "*Okay, we'll help you.*" So my husband Ernie came up also and they both helped me off the platform.

I guess the blind gentleman heard me scuffing along the church corridor after the service. So he asked his wife what was wrong with me. She came up and politely asked Ernie what was the matter. My husband told her I had Multiple Sclerosis, that it was getting progressively worse, and that I was sort of in the latter stages of this disease. Ernie also told her the next step for me would probably be to go into a wheelchair.

The man's wife went back and told her husband what my husband had said to her. As it turned out the next week, that gentleman came up to my husband in church and said that I didn't need to be sick anymore.

That blind gentleman's name, I would later find out, was Bill Irwin. Bill told my husband that he thought he could help me. He invited Ernie and me to visit his home so we could talk some more.

When we went to see Bill he said, "*If you really listen to me, and you really understand what I'm trying to tell you, you can get better.*" I listened to what Bill had to say.

51

Bill didn't seem to me to be just a "day-to-day" person. He just seemed to be very knowledgeable. When he spoke, he was very polished. I also respected him because I'd heard that he walked the Appalachian Trail blind, with his Seeing-Eye dog. He sounded as if he really knew what he was talking about.

Bill then explained what he wanted me to do. He suggested baby steps at first, which included juicing some carrots and drinking a green powder drink everyday called Barley Max. He warned me that it didn't taste too good, but suggested that I drink anywhere from 3-4 glasses of that each day ... spread throughout the day.

My first reaction to what Bill told us was, "*What do I have to lose?*" I'd tried everything else, and nothing worked. I'd tried medicines and psychologists. So why not give this a try?

I told Bill I was on lots of medications. He said that was okay. I also told him that I needed those medications in order to stay better. And Bill said, "*Take things as they come.*"

So that's what I began doing. Ernie bought a juicer and did the juicing for me. And I started drinking juiced carrots and Barley Max. After that, we never looked back!

At first, I still maintained my old diet, but just incorporated the juicing into it. I started feeling like I had a little more energy. Not a lot, but I did feel a change. Bill talked with Ernie some more, and after awhile, suggested that instead of continuing with baby steps that I just go straight ahead and fully change my diet. He recommended this because the disease had progressed so much.

Bill asked me if I was willing to do this. I told him I was. So he then told me I had to get all dairy and meat products out of my life. He said I shouldn't consume any animal based products ... anything that originated from a mother or father. Then he said I needed to get rid of caffeinated coffee, white flour and anything else that wasn't healthy.

Ernie was very supportive. He was willing to do this diet with me. So our home became a vegan-vegetarian one, instead of one serving the Standard American Diet. We arranged our meals so that about 85% of what we ate was raw. Even now, this is the ratio we still consume. We eat very few cooked meals.

"I Can't Explain It, But I Just Feel Good"

Exactly 4 months after beginning to do this, I got up about 5:30 am one morning. I felt like I had energy. Ernie asked me what was wrong. I said, "*I feel good.*" He replied, "*What do you mean you feel good?*" "*I can't explain it, but I just feel good ... I have energy,*" I answered.

"*Wow ... what do you want to do?*" my husband asked. So I said, "*Maybe later on today we can take a little walk. I haven't been for a walk outside in a long time. So let's take a walk.*"

Later that day, Ernie and I went outside. I started out by going to the end of our driveway. The AFO support the doctors had given me to wear on my foot, to prop it up and keep it from dragging, didn't feel comfortable. So I took it off.

It was then that I noticed my foot wasn't sagging. It wasn't just hanging anymore. I walked a little further and said to Ernie, "*I feel better without that.*" We put the AFO support away in the closet that day. I still have it in there.

I called Bill up afterwards and said, "*You know, I don't want to jump the gun here, but I want you to know that I gave up that AFO support on my foot because it wasn't comfortable anymore.*" And Bill said, "*Well, that's good.*"

About a week later, I said to Ernie, "*You know, I'm not having those visual symptoms ... or those awful cluster headaches.*" He said, "*Yeah, I've noticed that. If you're not having any cluster headaches then we don't need this great big tank of oxygen in here.*"

53

So I stopped the deliveries of the oxygen because the cluster headaches were gone.

So now there were 2 big symptoms of the disease that had gone away. As I got better, I was able to let go of certain medications the doctors had given me because the symptoms were no longer there. For example, when those things that felt like electric shocks in my legs went away, I no longer needed to take Amitriptyline when I went to bed because I no longer had pain.

Ernie would say to me, "*I can't believe this.*" And I'd say the same thing. I'd say, "*How can it be that just eating differently helps me, when after all of those years, nothing else helped?*" And he said, "*You know, I'm thinking a lot of it really does have to do with diet.*"

Again, I started to see these big changes after about 4 months of being on a mostly raw food diet. Up to that point, I didn't seem to notice much change. But all of a sudden, it was as if I had to get used to living in a healthy body again. I'd almost forgotten what it was to live years ago. I noticed all improvements because they felt great.

I was eventually able to give up all 11 medicines that I'd been taking. I slowly dropped them, one by one, because the symptoms were no longer there. I kept on thinking, "*Lord, I hope this doesn't return.*" That thought kept going on in my mind. So I asked Bill if I would ever go back to the way I was. He said, "*No ma'am, you won't go back that way unless you eat that way.*"

"My Life Was Completely Changed"

After being on my new diet for about a year, and feeling better, my husband and I decided to go to Baxter State Park here in Maine one day. Ernie encouraged me to walk into the woods a little bit and cross a brook. Then he asked if I wanted to take a little climb up the mountain. I said, "*I feel like it.*" And so he said, "*Let's try it.*"

We climbed 2300 feet into the air. It was snowing up on top a little bit. I called Bill from the top of that mountain and said, *"You're not going to believe where I am!"* That was my first mountain climb after getting well. It's still hard for me to believe that I lived in such a sick body for so many years.

My life was completely changed, as well as my husband's daily routine. Ernie didn't have to take care of me anymore, and he discovered that I could now do all the things he once had to do for me.

I was now able to go grocery shopping again. I was now able to take care of paying household bills. I even had to re-learn how to keep a checkbook. It had been so long since I'd kept one, and my mind hadn't been able to process some of the simple things necessary in order to keep it.

"I Had Another MRI Done"

After completely changing to my new diet, there weren't any foods I longed for that I'd eaten in the past. My new foods seemed to be nutritious. They seemed to be filling. And I just knew the old processed foods weren't good for my body. I'd learned that this new way of eating was healing to my body -- and the old way wasn't. So why would I go back to something that hurt my body?

There was actually a fear that if I ate those old foods that I'd go back to having symptoms. So I was happy not to eat them. Bill told me that, in a sense, this was almost like alcoholism. If a recovering alcoholic goes back to just one drink, they can fall back into alcoholism once again. But if they stay away from it then they won't crave it. So as long as I never picked up a bag of potato chips I'd never desire them again.

After I learned how to treat my body right, I didn't have any more cravings for the old foods. But I can still enjoy things like sweets. I can go into my freezer and get a frozen banana, blend it with my processor, and it comes out like ice cream. Then I put fresh strawberries and blueberries on top … or a little 100% maple syrup with walnuts, or pecans on top … and then I enjoy a wonderful sweet treat.

Very often, I put things like blueberries into the freezer and then take them out in the afternoon and enjoy them frozen. I do that with grapes too.

When I share the idea about eating raw with anyone I can usually tell less than 10 minutes into the conversation whether or not they're going to accept it. For some people, even though eating this way may be a cure for them, they're still going to be skeptical.

There are people who saw me very sick in the past, and know that I'm well now, who still can't apply this to their life. According to them, it's too strict of a regimen to follow. It's too much for them. They want a pill that's going to make them better. They don't want to work for the results. I had to work to get where I am. I couldn't take a pill and get better. The medicines never made me any better; they simply masked the symptoms.

What I try and offer people is an open door that can make them completely healthy again. And it's not just with diet, but through other choices also. You can't just have a good diet but also have stress and anger and frustration in your life and still be healthy. You have to make healthy choices in those areas too.

Being healthy is kind of like a circle. I would tell skeptics that if they want something to make them healthy then they have to be committed to this. It has to be something they really want.

I really, really wanted to get better. I'm sure other people want to get better, but they need to know that they can often get better without drugs and stay healthy.

As of right now, I'm in great shape. I just had some surgery on my shoulder because I fell and injured it during one of my mountain climbs. I had a minor shoulder repair.

According to my doctor, I'm doing about 3 times better than somebody that isn't in as good of shape as I am because they're not as healthy as I am. So he is really pleased with my progress.

My neurologist was skeptical about my progress against MS at first. She didn't want me to get my hopes up. But I discussed with her what I was going to do with the diet before I did it. After 2 years into my health change, she noticed such a difference in the gait of my walk that she decided to do another MRI on my brain. That was in 2004.

That MRI showed just 4 lesions on my brain. So at that time, my neurologist wouldn't say that my disease was "cured," but that I now had control over it, instead of it having control over me. She also noted on her report that I was consuming carrot juice and had changed the way I was eating. She also said that at this point she would no longer recommend any more treatment specifically for MS.

Just recently, before going into the hospital for shoulder surgery, I had another MRI done. This most recent MRI showed no lesions on my brain at all. So it appears as if all of the lesions I once had have now healed.

My neurologist hasn't seen this most recent scan yet. But I'm going to see her in a few weeks. I think she is going to be shocked. What doctors would now say about my condition is that the MS has been "arrested."

I have all the medical documents that prove this account. It's hard to describe the emotions I now feel as a healthy person ... now, after once being so sick. If you could have seen me at the peak of me being sick you would never have believed that my condition could ever turn around. There were days when my husband didn't think I'd make it through the day.

My husband and I climb 6 mountains a year now. We're living my life to the fullest. I'm so pleased that my story will be read. If just one person reads it and gets better then it'll be well worth it.

6
An Interview with Karen Hood
Testimony of Healing from Lupus

In 1973, when I was 19 yrs old, I woke up paralyzed on my right side. I was totally paralyzed on this side of my body, including the muscles on my face.

I ended up being in the hospital for almost 3 months. Then I had to use a wheelchair so I could get around for awhile afterwards.

After that initial paralyzation, I began to recover. I remember them giving me steroids and other medications, along with physical therapy. When I left the hospital after 3 months I was walking. I was a little weak and had a cane, but I was eventually able to start into physical fitness.

My condition was never diagnosed at the time. Doctors couldn't figure out what had caused it. The best guess offered to my condition was that it was possibly multiple sclerosis or a stroke. But it wasn't definitive because there were no MRIs available at that time.

For many years I never knew what had been wrong with me. But after developing that paralysis, I decided to go on a health regime. I stopped eating most meat and began feeling better. This diet change helped me lose weight. And I also started running 3 to 4 miles a day. I've stayed with this active lifestyle my whole life since then.

I wanted to be proactive with my health. A big part of this was trying to make sure that whatever had happened to me didn't happen again. Eventually, I went back to college to finish my degree. Then I went to law school and began my legal career afterwards.

"A Chronic Cough ... Severe Arthritis ... and Heart Palpitations"

I felt as if I was in total remission from that sickness until about 1997. It was then that I developed a chronic cough. Once again, it seemed as if nobody could diagnose the problem. But finally, after seeing about 12 doctors, I went up to the University of Michigan and was diagnosed with Lupus related lung disease.

The doctors there also told me that my paralyzation back in 1973 was when the Lupus probably set into my system. There had just been no way to diagnose it because the technology had not progressed to that point yet.

So I had no symptoms again until developing this chronic cough. I felt as if I'd been exceptionally healthy. But with lung trouble, I felt like things were really getting serious. The lupus had come out of remission and was beginning to wreak havoc over my life.

When I was diagnosed with Lupus, I was devastated ... but also relieved. It's really something being sick and not knowing what is the matter. So I was relieved, in that at least it was treatable. Being diagnosed with certain chronic diseases is no longer a death sentence today.

The doctors always prescribed medicine for my condition ... lots of medicine. So I began a number of treatments with medication. The chronic cough was abated somewhat, but the lupus continued attacking my body and other symptoms began appearing. Two of them were severe arthritis and heart palpitations. That's when I started thinking I really had to do something different in order to recover my health.

"This Diet Change Appears To Have Reversed My Condition"

About 12 years ago, I began eating macrobiotically. I felt like that helped me feel better. But even before I had started eating macrobiotically, I had read about a mostly raw food diet promoted by a man named George Malkmus. I thought about going to his center, which he'd named Hallelujah Acres, in order to learn more about a raw food diet.

I didn't go at that time though because I felt like such a diet was too boring. I felt as if raw food couldn't be prepared to be very tasty. I thought it was just about eating apples and salads everyday. I didn't understand that there was a lot of creativity in the things that you can do with raw food to make it interesting. So I decided to go with the macrobiotics at the time because there was a lot of cooked food and ways to prepare things.

Last year though, when the heart palpitations came upon me, I had to go into the hospital. The staff wanted to give me 6 more medications to take ... things like Lipitor, and other drugs. But I said, "*No, I can't do that!*" The thoughts came back to me once again about visiting Hallelujah Acres.

I ended up going to a *Hallelujah Acres Retreat Center* in Plant City, Florida. While there, I had a hands-on experience with raw foods for a whole week. I just loved it. I've been doing it ever since.

I didn't approach this like I was going to try and use diet in place of modern medicine, but in addition to modern medicine. I realize that somebody who has had the level of sickness that I've had may have to be on medication. But I wanted this to be as minimal as possible.

This means that sometimes I've had to fight with my doctors, and we've gone back and forth about certain things. But ultimately, I respect their knowledge, realizing that I didn't go to medical school. But sometimes we do have a back and forth exchange.

Taking 16 medications at one time was horrible. It was very depressing. First of all, you're a slave to medication when you have to take it like that. Even though it's a blessing to have medications on one hand, the whole process takes a lot of time and attention. Using 3 inhalers, opening bottles every 3 hours, taking pills at bedtime for this and that ... it can drive you crazy.

Now things are so different. I don't even use the inhalers anymore. When you eat mostly raw, and practice juicing, then your body just responds to it because it's like nature's healthy medicine.

This diet change appears to have reversed my condition. I've not had heart palpitations for awhile. The chronic cough has disappeared. And the progression of the other symptoms I've had from Lupus – such as the arthritis – has slowed. I still have arthritis. But I also feel like I'm "working on it."

Specifically, I've had problems with Lupus related rheumatoid arthritis. This is one area where I've kept using medication up to this point because I tried to get through without it and it wasn't possible. Then again, a lot of this takes time. I've seen so many improvements ... in so many areas. And I haven't seen things getting any worse!

It seems as if I've rapidly improved in some areas, but the arthritis is improving at a snail's pace. So, depending upon what area you talk about, this is how I've experienced things.

I changed my diet in January of 2008 and I've been able to get down to 4 medications, down from the 16 that I had during the height of 2007. In 2007, I went into the hospital 4 times. The last hospital visit lasted 3 weeks. The doctors suspected that I had blood clots in my lungs from the Lupus. But in 2008, I didn't spend one second in the hospital. Now, it's 2009, and I'm still doing well.

61

I feel pretty healthy right now. I've had so many areas of healing in my body that I'm simply waiting for the arthritis to go away too.

My body feels like it's getting better and stronger everyday. And now I know we have a part to play that goes beyond just food. For example, I exercise everyday. You have to exercise.

"Anyone Who Is Skeptical About Eating This Way Should Do Some Research"

I've always been an advocate of trying to use diet as a way to improve my health because in my background growing up, my family didn't tend to have a lot of raw fruits and vegetables around. I grew up eating things like collard greens cooked in grease. I've always believed we shouldn't eat like that.

Now I really love eating healthy. I love my carrot juice. I love my salads and I really get excited over this way of eating.

When I attended the raw food retreat in Florida, I was already eating macrobiotically. So it wasn't a big jump to start eating a mostly raw, totally vegan diet. I made the change the very first day I was there. And I've never gone back. I eat about 75% raw and 25% cooked food everyday.

There are 2 things I do miss about the way I used to eat. I miss salmon and also fried fish. Being a vegan now, I eat a 100% plant-based diet. But I used to love fish so much I had it almost every day.

That helped me to discover something amazing though … that I could be on a macrobiotic diet, and still have high cholesterol. When I came out of the hospital in 2007, I discovered my cholesterol was high.

About 3 months after going all-vegan, my cholesterol was so low that I had to make sure my doctor knew that I hadn't been taking Lipitor to reduce it. My cholesterol became low because of the change to a raw diet. It's even lower now. So this diet has been a real blessing.

I constantly take food preparation classes because preparing raw dishes can be labor intensive. It does take some energy. But it really works. The juicing really works … and the whole raw eating program I learned at Hallelujah Acres. I feel as if anyone who consumes a living diet, yet doesn't have any serious illness, is being proactive with their health.

There is nothing negative I could say about eating this way. For me, the experience has been all good. Anyone who is skeptical about eating this way should do some research. I think they'd find, just based upon their research, that there is nothing to lose. The only thing that could happen is that there could be a positive impact on their life … both physically and mentally. There are a lot of mental benefits to eating this way as well.

I still go to see my main doctor every 3 months. I go quarterly. All of my doctors are amazed at how well I'm doing now. They are also thrilled about my improvement. They've been very receptive to the information I bring them.

I would tell anyone who is considering this kind of diet in an effort to change their health, "*Just do it!*" Be willing to make the sacrifice to just do it.

I'd also suggest that they find someone to assist them in learning how to prepare their raw foods in new ways. They'll discover that when they combine right eating with exercise, they're almost guaranteed to see some type of improvement in their health. Even if they don't experience a full cure, they need to see progressive sickness may not be the norm. An improvement in health makes it all worthwhile.

7

"In ~~God~~ Doctors I Trust"

We all operate by a certain degree of "faith" in life. Even if you don't consciously hold to a religious faith per se, you operate with a certain level of faith or "trust" in the way the world works. This includes how you relate to others, how you conduct your business, and to whom you seek out help when it's needed.

If you want to pay your electric bill by sending a check to the utility company then you put one in the mail after writing it out and trust the workers in the postal system are going to get it to where it needs to go. Whenever you get behind the wheel of a car you place a certain amount of trust in the likelihood that other drivers on the road are going to follow traffic laws and drive responsibly, including staying in their lanes so their cars won't collide with your vehicle. Etc.

This is what I mean when I say you exercise a certain amount of faith in those around you everyday. And this trust factor is especially present when you go to a doctor for help in diagnosing a physical problem so you can then receive a prescription to get well.

In other words, we all have faith or trust in both persons and processes. This is no less true when it comes to the subject of diet and health. Your ability to wade through various opinions in search of the truth will be affected by your worldview.

Whom do you believe, for example, when one doctor suggests that diet can dramatically impact health ... but another says diet probably isn't very important at all when dealing with most diseases? How will you weigh various opinions, especially when even scientifically trained medical physicians aren't in agreement? You may want to find out where your doctor(s) stand on these issues.

We take it for granted that medical doctors are both intelligent and highly trained professionals. And I would certainly agree that is true. But you may want to ask yourself if the words of every doctor should be taken "by faith" as a pronouncement of absolute, omniscient truth.

I once read that for many individuals, the term "MD" stands for "My Deity." And it does sometimes seem our modern culture ascribes an almost god-like reverence towards physicians. The workings of the body are such a mystery to most of us. We naturally want to convey a high respect towards those who seemingly understand those mysteries to a certain degree.

But doctors are certainly not infallible. And neither are all the things that take place within hospitals and patient treatment centers across the country. Mortal men and women sometimes make mistakes … however well intentioned their actions.

Getting Sick While Trying to Get Well

The term "iatrogenic" refers to an *unwanted* condition that is brought about by a physician or a medical procedure. It is estimated that as many as 200,000 people die every year in the U.S. as a result of iatrogenic causes.[14]

Dr. Barbara Starfield of the Dept. of Health Policy and Management at Johns Hopkins University was once quoted as saying that deaths resulting from iatrogenic reasons are the 3rd largest cause of death in the U.S. That means only heart disease and cancer kills more people (although it's not usually on any health statistic charts with these diseases).

She once estimated:

7,000 people die each year from medical errors in hospitals

12,000 die each year from unnecessary surgery

20,000 die from "other" iatrogenic errors

80,000 die from infections acquired in hospitals

106,000 die from the negative affects of drugs administered to them by doctors[15]

Such statistics are well known in the medical community. But most hospital patients have never seen figures that indicate the large amount of these kinds of problems.

"Indeed, a study done in the early 1980s by the U.S. Health Care Financing Administration showed that, for patient medication alone, the average hospital had a 12 percent error rate. A decade later, things had not improved: According to a Harvard University study, 10% of all cardiac arrests in hospitals are attributable to medication errors. Errors in the medicine patients receive can occur for a variety of reasons. However, a book entitled Medication Errors: Causes and Prevention by two Temple University pharmacology professors, Michael Cohen and Neil Davis, attributes much of the problem to the mindless deference given the "boss" of the patient's case: the attending physician. According to Professor Cohen, "in case after case, patient's nurses, pharmacists, and other physicians do not question the prescription."[16]

The above should encourage you, at the very least, to consider all options before blindly accepting prescribed treatments. Always ask your doctor questions. Have procedures and medicines fully explained to you.

For example, such questions may include: "What is the rate of success (and failure) related to these procedures and drugs?" "Are there any related side effects?" "Will the drugs being prescribed negatively react with any other drugs I'm currently taking?"

You also may want to ask what the percentages of success are regarding the treatments being prescribed to you. Are they 90% successful ... 60% ... 40% ... 25% ... less? Wouldn't you agree this is good for you to know?

Asking questions is important, especially considering the options typically offered to patients who are fighting serious diseases. For example, there are 3 basic ways the medical community currently treats cancer:

Drugs. Drugs are often toxic to the body and they're often used to simply suppress symptoms, not deal with the causes of disease. Hundreds of thousands of people die around the world each year because of prescription medications.

Surgery. Cutting unwanted things out of the body is a common treatment. But simply cutting out problems, such as tumors or other masses, never deals with the issue of "why" they formed in the first place. This doesn't mean having surgery is wrong. It simply means that when used as a remedy for diseases most surgeries never deal with any reasons why the conditions warranting surgery happened in the first place.

Radiation. Radiation is often used in cancer treatment. It is akin to "burning" out cancerous cells. The problem, of course, is that this process doesn't just kill cancerous cells; it kills healthy cells too. There are no properties of healing in radiation; radiation is about killing unwanted cells.

Despite incredible advances in medical technology over recent years in the areas of diagnosis and surgery, these 3 basic ways for treating cancer are still in place: drugs, surgery and radiation.

You may also note those approaches are big moneymakers for the medical establishment. While I believe everyone is entitled to make a profit through his or her work, you should be aware that financial incentives may be in play when it comes to how you will be medically treated.

It's your right to question prescribed medical treatments. After all, it's your health. You're also going to be responsible for the bills incurred. The bigger issue is about fully understanding your treatment options – along with any risks involved.

The fact that drugs, surgery and radiation are "accepted" medical treatments for treating cancer and other diseases doesn't mean they're automatically "best." It simply means those are the best ones available right now for medically treating the disease. One question to ask though is whether or not other options may be available – such as a nutritional approach.

Important Note: Remember, if you're currently taking any physician prescribed medication you shouldn't change or alter any medications without the assistance of a physician.

Has Your Doctor Studied Nutrition?

When it comes to the subject of diseases, it seems as if the very same medical schools that are often so good at teaching doctors how to save the lives of trauma victims often neglect to sufficiently address how (or even if) the human body can heal itself through proper nutrition.

Many doctors haven't studied diet and its connection to disease in-depth. Nor have many physicians ever taken a single professional course on nutrition. Why is this?

The fact some diseases, such as cancer, are much more common in certain parts of the world than others should encourage the whole medical community to ask why there are far fewer reported instances in some places than in others. In general, cancer rates are much lower in parts of the world where meat and dairy consumption is very low.

If you ask most American doctors whether or not there is a connection between a disease like cancer and diet you'll get a whole range of opinions. Many don't seem to connect the disease with diet at all. And few seem to say the body can heal itself of cancer simply through a change in diet. A limited number of physicians are now treating cancer using a holistic approach, along with conventional medicine.

Since the practice of medicine is a heavily regulated enterprise, medical doctor(s) may have genuine concerns about deviating from conventional treatment methods in favor of more holistic approaches. At this present time, there is no sign the medical community in western nations is going to change from its current approaches to disease treatment.

Instead of using the human body as a chemistry experiment, however, the medical establishment might benefit by shifting more focus to nutritional biology. The research linking nutrition and health are now stronger than ever. But they're not emphasized enough.

Maybe this is because most patients "want to have their cake and eat it too." Maybe too few of us want to hear about changing our diet in order to get healthy? But if getting well meant simply changing your present eating habits then would you be willing to at least give it a try?

Keep in mind that doctors suffer with the same disease and cancer rates as the rest of the population. They're no healthier than the population as a whole. And despite the hundreds of millions of dollars spent on things such as cancer research there are more people in the West dying of cancer and suffering from chronic diseases today than ever before.

8
An Interview with Suzy Hoseus
Testimony of Healing
from Bipolar & Depression

I'm a stay at home mom who lives in Kentucky with my family. My husband and I have 3 children and I presently homeschool the younger two.

My story about bipolar disorder began in childhood. There was a lot of stress in my life growing up. My parents divorced when I was young. And my stepfather was an alcoholic.

There were also other traumas. I had 10 root canals and 10 caps put on my teeth when I was 17 years old. My sister died when I was 18. There were also 5 deaths of others who were close to me within one year. So there was a lot of trauma in my young life. This stress affected every area of my being; it touched emotional, chemical and physical areas.

Before anyone ever suggested I had what is called "bipolar disorder," I experienced 3 years of what is known as "cycling." These were periods when I went into deep, dark depression and then manic, sleepless episodes for months at a time. Then I would come out of it. So things would cycle up and down and any period could last up to 6 months at a time.

About 3 years into this period of cycling, I'd been to different doctors and universities, and I knew something was terribly wrong. I didn't know anything about "bipolar" and wasn't even aware there was a label for what I was experiencing. One day a friend said to me, "*Suzy, I think you're suffering from manic depression.*" That just hit me like a bullet. I thought, "*Wow, that is exactly what this is.*" I just had never heard a label for it.

When I finally discovered it was a medical condition I considered it a blessing because at least I finally knew what was wrong. It was a profound relief to be able to at least give it a label.

The various doctors I continued to see told me I'd have this condition for my whole life and also that I'd have to be on medications for the rest of my life. They felt it was just the way things were.

"I Just Felt Hopeless"

Over the next 20 years I saw many different doctors. I went through psychotherapy and received confirmation that this indeed was bipolar. I was again informed that I'd have to be on medications and there was no hope for me to ever get off the medications.

The medications allowed me to get a type of pseudo-sleep. But I never dreamed or experienced a natural type of sleep by any means. The drugs just knocked me out.

I was very dependent upon medication. Any time I tried to get off the medication I'd go through an episode of severe depression, have to be hospitalized, then I'd have to start all over again. So I really felt trapped.

There were periods during this 20-year span that I fell into desperation. I felt that if this were going to be the quality of my life then I'd always be in despair. I just didn't know there was any other way to deal with this other than what the doctors told me. I was just so indoctrinated with the belief that I'd have to be on medications for the rest of my life that there were times I just felt hopeless.

Apart from drugs, the only other thing that was really prescribed for my condition was psychotherapy. During my 20+ years of depression I had a slew of different psychiatrists and counselors. I guess that was just a part of protocol for treatment.

I can only begin to guess how much it cost for all the drugs and the psychotherapy treatment I was given. There is no way to assess the total cost of the thousands upon thousands of dollars spent, along with endless hours of treatment sessions and hospital stays. The really sad part about this is that I regard much of the treatment I was given as potentially harmful if not counterproductive.

I did become somewhat close to a couple of therapists I had in the sense that there was a real relationship bond. Those 2 gentlemen helped bring me to some level of healing, but they were somewhat unconventional in their practice. Their teachings took me "out of the box" from what I'd mostly experienced with conventional treatment methods. For the most part, nobody was really hitting upon the problem.

In my opinion, the treatments prescribed to me never dealt with the root cause of my illness. In my situation, my body was depleted of certain nutrients that enabled my brain to function properly. And my brain was also so drug laden with toxins it wasn't able to function properly either. When the mixes of chemical additives, plus poor behavior choices on my part were added together, I now see these were things that were never addressed.

"Full Time Healing"

After about 10 years into the 20-year span I started getting into nutrition as a way to possibly help my condition and deal with this illness. I'd change my diet, got off some medications and felt like I was doing better. But I didn't realize this would bring on what I now know as "a healing crisis," where the healing process could include relapses that were actually part of the healing.

I'd never really acquired a full picture of natural health until I lived in Florida. It was there I heard a speaker named George Malkmus talk about health and nutrition. I learned about juicing and also that deliberate, intense nutritional action can be taken to improve one's health. It was then I also realized those healing crises I'd experienced were a part of the actual healing process.

When I first heard George speak I didn't feel I was ready to make that full jump into a complete change in diet. But it did plant a seed in me. The idea to change my diet had been planted earlier on. But about 6 months after hearing him speak I experienced what I thought may be a very serious health problem one day. I really thought I was dying. That is what really got my attention and prompted me to fully change the way I ate.

I called a friend who practices naturopathy and he suggested that I fast for 3 days. I told him that I couldn't fast for 3 days because of my medication. But by this time I'd already started eating cooked rice and vegetables, so I was no longer on what may be termed the "Standard American Diet."

But now I was ready for the "leap of faith" and embraced a mostly raw diet. When I did that my body started to detoxify itself immediately and at a rapid rate. There were days when my body would develop cysts and eliminate puss. My skin color would change. I felt very sick and was pretty much laid up for about 9 months after starting to do this. I quit my job and let my body go into full-time healing.

I stuck with the diet because I knew what was going on in my body. I had started studying a correspondence course curriculum by Joel Robbins, M.D. (from the Health and Wellness Clinic, and founder of the College of Natural Health).

When my body would go through a new healing crisis, I learned that sometimes doing everything right can make you feel sick for awhile. Sickness can happen when your body is detoxifying, but it's actually a part of the healing process. The stricter I got with my diet the more my body would detox.

Dr. Robbins has a gift for taking complicated material and turning it into really simple and straightforward ideas. He broke down anatomy and physiology and nutrition in various sections of his curriculum in a way that was very tangible for me. Those ideas really helped me. If I hadn't known what was going on when it came to detoxification then I probably would have just assumed I should go into a hospital or something.

I later came to see that when I'd started down the path of nutrition 10 years earlier I would start to get well, but go through a healing crisis, and then somebody like my mother would take me back to get more of the old treatment. I mean, there were times I'd be locked up and injected with drugs against my will.

I saw the change in my lifestyle and diet to all-natural living foods as my ticket out of chronic depression and manic episodes. I believed in it. And I believe God called me to a life of Whole Health.

I remember being outside one particular day during this time of healing. The temperature was 70 degrees and the weather was perfect. It was one day that I actually felt pretty good, which was rare. I had been praying and I felt like the Lord just said to me, "*Suzy, I'm going to bless you with more children.*" I was 39 at the time and had been previously told after my son's birth that I should never even consider having more children. (Doctors told me I would be too high of a risk.)

A year or so later I got pregnant. I just knew it was going to be a girl and that we would call her Leah. Leah's homebirth when I was 40 went exceptionally well. At 43, I got pregnant again and knew Ben and Leah's sister's name would be Lindsay. She was also home-birthed and in both instances, I experienced no postpartum depression.

"If You Want True Healing ..."

My advice to anyone who is thinking about doing a lifestyle and diet change like this is to be very careful about who you seek counsel. There are major differences of opinion between an allopathic doctor, a naturopath, and/or a Natural Hygienist.[17]   Organizations such as Hallelujah Acres or Earth Save can provide information on educated and enlightened individuals.

It's extremely difficult to get off of psychotropic medications.   Unlike most other disease processes, you're primarily dealing with the brain. This can be devastatingly frightening at times.   It's not like most other diseases.   I distrusted myself at times because I had been sick for so long.

It's not like going through just physical pain.   With bipolar disorder you go through emotional pain, torment, and anxiety. There is much to learn in handling these severe emotions.

I'd go through a healing crisis and think to myself, "*This was exactly why I took up medications.*" Or I'd think, "*This is exactly why I took an anti-anxiety med ... this is exactly why I took a sleeping pill.*" And yet, by the grace of God, I was able to withstand the symptoms.   It was intense.

If I had called a regular medical doctor during that time, he or she probably would have told me that I needed to go to the hospital or go back on medication.   For example, I endured periods of intense insomnia because I had depended upon sleeping medication for 20 years. So I had to overcome it.

I've learned through sharing with other people who try to travel this road that they too get into jams and it's tough to not rely on medications.   A person going through a time like this needs to be able to call somebody who is knowledgeable and be provided appropriate encouragement and support to help them get through a temporary period of discomfort.

There are times when you have to go through discomfort. You have to go through the pain towards the reward. *PAIN* has become my acronym for: *Patience-Appreciation-Insight-Newness.* You have to be patient and go through discomfort. You have to thank God for the time of healing … and having the insight to realize that you have to go through it. This is what I have found to be the healing and transformation process.

Deciding to change your lifestyle and the way you eat in order to acquire Whole Health is a choice. A lot of it comes down to faith. Skepticism is a choice that can keep people in the dark. Some people I know think I'm so extreme on how I eat and live. But they've never eaten raw or lived the way I do. So how can they suggest I'm off base when they don't know anything about it?

Anyone can be skeptical if they want to be. But they should ask if their skepticism is going to be beneficial in light of what they want. If you want true healing, and if you want Whole Health, then seek God for truth in what brings optimal health and vitality.

"I Haven't Even Had An Aspirin Since the Year 2000"

It's been 10 years now since my healing and I haven't even had an aspirin since the year 2000. I'm in mostly excellent health. I still have some extra weight in my stomach though, where I carry my emotions. My digestive system still isn't where I want it to be. But I do exceptionally well considering that I'm raising 3 kids, teaching seminars and promoting my book while my husband travels frequently. He is the author of a best-selling book called, *"Toyota Culture,"* and travels worldwide.

My life is completely different now ... as far as stress levels go. I feel very charmed to be able to be at home raising my children and feeling especially blessed that I have an awesome teenage son who helps me with the two little girls we now have.

We have a large house and in the winters, I get up in the morning, build a fire, water the plants, feed the animals and kids, and then homeschool. I'm still learning how to relax. But I'm not now where I'm going to be.

I think that one of the biggest blessings now is just being able to sleep and wake up rested. This includes having clarity of mind, crispness, and true energy, while also enjoying an improved memory. I had been to a point where there was much harm done to me by all the different medications ... especially the sleep medications.

The fact I'm able to do all I do now without medications, or any hard-core symptoms of depression, is a miracle. The sickness I endured requires lots of love for healing. Sometimes I think the food part can be emphasized too much.

I've been very blessed. I have a husband and children now who really love me. I bathe in this love. That has got me through as much as any energy I get from all the physical components of health. My family has really supported me. That is a key component for healing, especially when dealing with a disorder like bipolar. Much healing needs to take place and bridges need to be made from years of hurt and struggle.

The first couple of years I was on a raw diet program, my husband and son would juice 8-10 glasses of vegetable juice in the morning for me everyday. And to this day, my son will get up and juice 3-5 green juices for me. He does that before he goes to school because he knows how beneficial it is.

This is the kind of support that I enjoy from my family. It's a big reason why I've been so blessed. And it's why I want to extend myself, as I'm able, to help others.

. . . .

Suzy Hoseus is a wife, mother and author of *Healing Bipolar and Depression: My Journey to Whole Health*. To find out more about this book and Suzy's story, visit her website at www.lifelearningministries.org

9

An Interview with Lee Jernigan
Testimony of Recovery from Brain Cancer

I own a local business called First General Services. It's part of a national company based in Fort Lauderdale, Florida that does insurance repair work. Our team specializes in cost-effective remodeling for both residential and commercial properties that have been damaged by smoke, fire or mold.

Around 1999 a pastor friend of mine named Horace went on what is known as the Hallelujah Diet. He told stories whenever we'd get together about how he and a nutritionist were now teaching others about eating mostly raw foods. Horace said he was seeing individuals experience reversal of many kinds of diseases by adopting this new way of eating.

I had a lot of confidence in Horace. I didn't think he would ever embellish a story just to impress me. I trusted him as a person and the things he shared with me. I thought to myself, "*Wow, if I ever get really sick then I'll consider doing that too.*"

Horace is in his 60s. Before my cancer diagnosis I remembered asking him, "*If you could tell me the biggest thing this diet has done for you personally then what would it be?*" He said, "*Lee, I have more energy than I know what to do with.*"

My friend's words began to take up more of my thinking because I'd begun suffering what appeared to be sort of a "mental shutdown." I'd been feeling that way for several years. But then it began to get worse. I actually began thinking I wouldn't be able to function if it continued much longer.

In July of 2004 I lost one of my sisters to atrophy of the brain. She had been going downhill for about 15 years. Doctors couldn't figure out what was wrong with her. She'd gone to specialists and all anyone could ever tell us was that she had atrophy of the brain. Her doctors were never able to find out why.

My sister had gone from being totally independent to being completely cared for by my parents, then to a nursing home, then to having seizures, then into a coma and then passed ... she was only 43.

My other sister (the twin of my sister who died) then began having the same type of symptoms. We immediately brought her to the Medical College of Georgia also because they're known for doing cutting edge work in the area of neurology.

In November of 2004 I accompanied this sister when she went in for some testing. After they finished testing her I asked if they could also do a brain scan on me. Even though I didn't have the same symptoms that both of my sisters had experienced, such as equilibrium problems and shaking, I was constantly feeling mentally as if I were going down a dark hole.

I got to thinking that if I underwent a brain scan it would give physicians a baseline to compare against should other symptoms begin appearing. The doctor consented and performed an MRI on me.

The next day I received a phone call from the doctor and she said, "*We've found what looks to be a tumor in your brain Lee. You need to come in and talk to us.*" Both my wife and I were in shock.

We went in and met with doctors the next day. It turned out to be a malignant brain tumor. When the doctor said, "*Cancer,*" I hardly remembered anything else she talked about during the rest of that conversation.

There are various stages of brain cancer. Stage-1 is benign, stage-2 is malignant and eventually goes into final stage-4 and then death. Mine had been diagnosed as a stage-2 astrocytoma.

At that point the doctor, after consulting others, said my tumor was inoperable. But in the next 4 days we heard about a hospital in Texas named MD Anderson several times. So we sent our case out to Houston, Texas where MD Anderson is located. They are on the cutting edge of cancer treatments. They took my case.

"I Immediately Went On the Vegan Diet"

Upon being diagnosed with brain cancer I immediately went on the vegan diet I'd learned about from my friend Horace. I also stopped eating the things he said were harmful foods: meats, dairy products, white sugar, white flour, standard table salt and other refined foods.

I began studying nutrition diligently. One of the things I discovered was the importance of juicing. So I began juicing 64 ounces of carrot juice a day. That became an effort my whole family helped out with.

In the meantime, my wife and I began preparing to go down to Texas for brain surgery. I met with a neurosurgeon before the holidays and scheduled the date for January 12th of 2005.

All the way up to the time of surgery I continued with my new diet. I was beginning to feel awesome prior to having that procedure. My mental sharpness began picking up. And I began having lots of energy after about a month of eating this new way ... just as my friend Horace had experienced.

I really began to think I could beat this tumor without having any surgery whatsoever. My family really encouraged me to have it though. We talked it over and decided that if it were obvious the tumor had shrunk in size when they took a new MRI before the operation then I wouldn't move forward with it.

When the hospital in Texas took that MRI it showed the tumor was still the same size. It hadn't shrunk, but it hadn't increased in size either. So things proceeded as planned.

According to my doctors, the procedure went pretty well overall. My physicians released me from ICU just 2 days afterwards. My immediate recovery seemed to go pretty well too.

I'd wrongly assumed, however, the specialist at MD Anderson would be able to reach the area of the tumor without having to disturb other parts of my brain. That turned out to not be the case. The surgeons ended up moving my left frontal lobe to get to the affected area. It turns out this is now the area that causes my current physical and mental neurological challenges. For example, I tend to lose my train of thought easily nowadays.

During surgery my doctors took samples of the cancerous tissue, put them under a microscope and examined them. The pathologist called us about 2 weeks later and said the labeling index of the tissue was recorded as "very slow." When I asked one of my doctors what that meant he explained that any number under a "3" was considered to be a "slow growth" tissue.

The lowest number that doctor had ever seen was a "1." According to my pathology report, the sample from me was .5 or less -- which indicates my tumor hadn't been growing.

For most patients with brain tumors, the cancer continues to grow until seizures begin happening -- followed eventually by death. The specialist never tried to explain why the index for my tumor was so low. Before he left at the end of our meeting he looked at me and said, "*You are an exception!*"

That same doctor advised me to undergo chemo even though what was left of the tumor wasn't growing. I politely refused it. He eventually wrote a letter and dismissed me from being a patient under his care any longer. My issue with chemo is that I was concerned it would reverse what I was doing through diet, which was to supercharge my immune system to fight off the cancer. The chemo would only shrink the tumor some and only offered a 25% chance of working.

I feel like I'm getting better very slowly. My post-surgery physical condition has definitely improved. I know our bodies can self-heal because new cells over time replace old ones in every area of our bodies. That encourages me in the midst of my current physical and mental struggles.

The challenges I deal with now are mostly because of how the front area of my brain was altered by the surgery. That area affects energy, drive and initiative. It's a huge effort for me to get up and get moving everyday. It's also hard for me to multi-task right now. But I truly believe lots of prayer and this diet are what keep me going.

"Proper Nutrition Has Affected My Body"

Adopting this new diet has been very challenging. Before hearing I had cancer I honesty didn't think I'd ever be able to change to a vegan diet. But I discovered that when I came to a point of experiencing serious sickness and disease it changed my life.

Prior to changing my diet I regularly consumed lots of fast food. I'd always drive up to Wendy's for a burger on my way to the next job. I probably drank a pot of coffee everyday all by myself too.

Despite the health challenges of the past few years I feel as if I've been really blessed ... not just with physical recovery, but in other aspects of my life. My business employees have been super with regards to running most operations. There is no way I could've focused on both my contracting business and fighting this tumor. So I'm very grateful to them for their support.

Prior to my new diet I weighed about 218 pounds. That is heavy for a guy like me, who stands at 6' 1" in height. I lost weight immediately after adopting veganism. Now I try to stay around 180 pounds. I could easily go under that weight by eating more raw food, but I've chosen to eat more cooked food instead and keep my weight up.

It's very interesting to see how proper nutrition has affected my body in other ways. My hair is thicker. My nails grow in stronger than before. And my skin looks different and is tougher. I don't get nearly as winded when I exert myself either.

I saw a guy on Oprah once who worked with a group of women over a period of 6-8 weeks. The goal was for them to look younger by using diet as a tool instead of plastic surgery. After following the diet he prescribed to them those women looked as though they'd had plastic surgery.

One practical area of challenge is food preparation. There is a lot of preparation and a lot of learning with this lifestyle. My wife has picked up a lot of good ideas and incorporated them into her cooking for me.

I bought a VitaMix blender to help make some food preparation go faster. The VitaMix comes with a lot of recipes too. I can use it to make heated vegetable soups very easily. One particular recipe book I really like is called, "*How We All Went Raw*," by Charles, George Nungesser and Coralanne Nungesser.

I still eat a mostly raw diet. But I enjoy plenty of cooked foods as well. I consume things like steamed vegetables and stir fry with rice. I've also started eating things like guacamole, avocado and nuts such as walnuts, almonds and cashews. They're included to add more fat into my foods.

I also enjoy having some good things off the shelf such as toasted "Ezekiel Bread" with almond butter. There are many mornings when I enjoy homemade shakes that

84

include ingredients such as Flaxseed, Brewer's Yeast, rice milk and blueberries.

I'm beginning to enjoy green smoothies in the afternoons. Those are made with things like walnuts, apples, bananas, pineapple, collards, kale, spinach and ginger. They taste good and provide me with a wonderful energy boost.

"Better Pursuing Health This Way"

About six months after my surgery I met a man named Richard at an event for my children's school. This man is a father whose children began attending the same school as my kids after his family moved to our area from another state.

In 1997, Richard was diagnosed with brain cancer -- a stage-4 glioblastoma. His doctors were sure he was going to die. But he went ahead and had surgery, chemo and radiation. He is still very much alive though.

After his diagnosis he saw an herbalist and got on the same raw food diet that I'm now doing also. In hindsight, he wishes that he'd never had the chemo or radiation.

He juices everyday, eats mostly raw and also takes a dietary supplement he considers to be very helpful called "Juice Plus," which is a product that offers nutrients extracted from 17 different vegetables and fruits.

Every 6 months Richard sponsors an event in our locale where he brings in a doctor to speak about how certain foods can impact the body's health through proper nutrition. I've attended those lectures and enjoyed them very much. Richard has really been an encouragement to me.

I asked him if he knows of any other individual who has ever survived a stage-4 glioblastoma brain tumor and he said he has only heard of 3 others before him. It's almost unheard of.

The way I look at it is that if I continue eating this way there is a chance I'll live. I'm sure that if I had continued to eat a Standard American Diet I'd already be dead. I am pretty disciplined with my diet because I want to live.

I've found out that eating right, getting sunshine, exercise and having a Godly peace – all combined – can be very powerful. It's not good to be dependent upon medications. They might be good for a while ... to patch and manage difficult symptoms. But if you can slowly get your body and immune system built back up naturally then it's so much better pursuing health this way.

10

Are You Meant to Be a Carnivore or Herbivore?

The idea of consuming a diet that doesn't include meat (or many of the other items we discuss in this book) often sounds crazy to those who first hear about it. After all, hasn't man consumed meat for thousands of years?

History records the fact that animals have been hunted in order to provide mankind with nourishment for millennia. And as civilizations developed, animals such as cattle were specifically raised in order to supply meat for consumption within the limits and demands of managed market economies.

So what is the big deal with meat? That's a great question.

Before digging into a few details, let me first say that I personally don't have a moral problem with eating meat. I was raised to be a "meat and potatoes" kind of guy. I used to go hunting and fishing as a teenager. I'm not a member or supporter of the left-wing group PETA (People for the Ethical Treatment of Animals), which sees no difference between all animal life and human life.

Meat consumption, for me, doesn't have anything to do with a morality debate about whether or not it's wrong to raise chickens or kill a steer. It's simply about what is the healthiest thing to eat. Personal culinary preferences or moral stances over meat consumption don't have any bearing upon whether or not meat is a healthy thing to eat.

Western diet today isn't about pure survival as it was when mankind functioned as hunters and gatherers or was in the stages of early civilization. If you or a loved one want to eat healthy in this day and age then the primary issue is whether or not you'll be able to experience life to the fullest via a Standard Western Diet.

With that in mind, I do not now believe it's possible to eat meat in today's world without substantially increasing the risk of acquiring a host of debilitating diseases … especially cancer. I also believe it'll be very difficult for your body to heal itself of serious disease unless you stop eating meat (and other foods that may have caused the condition to begin with).

Some individuals (not many, but some) consume what most of us know as the Standard American Diet and go through life without too many physical problems. They don't get cancer. Nor do they experience an onslaught of other debilitating ailments, physical disabilities or chronic diseases. The question, however, is whether or not this is the rule rather than the exception.

Many scholars now believe that diseases such as cancer and others now commonplace in western civilization are frequently caused by what we put into our bodies. In recent conversations with cancer survivors who switched from a Standard American Diet to one of primarily "living foods," their cancer was either arrested or simply went away altogether after fundamentally changing their diet.

That doesn't mean the diet itself cured them. The theory here is that the body receives the nutrients necessary through proper diet to heal itself. In other words, the body's own self-healing functions kicked in and fought the disease in order to bring healing to the body.

Chemicals in the Meat

The issue goes beyond just the meat itself too. One prominent fact often overlooked by meat advocates is that the way meat is processed today as part of the food supply is far different than in previous generations.

Most of today's cattle and poultry are fed with products filled with harmful chemicals designed to add weight to the animals so they can produce more profit for the producers. Again, I have no problem whatsoever with the existence of a free "meat" market or anyone making profits from it. If that's what producers want to put into meat and consumers are willing to pay for it then fine. But that doesn't mean meat is healthy for us to consume.

If the marketplace wants to pay for and eat these products then it's their right to do so. But most of the marketplace doesn't know how carcinogenic (cancer-causing) today's meat and other animal-based products (including the chemicals and steroids they're produced with) can be to the human body.

Are you meant to be a carnivore (meat eater)?

"And God said, Behold, I have given you every herb bearing seed, which is upon the face of all the earth, and every tree, in which is the fruit of a tree yielding seed; to you it shall be for meat (food)." Genesis 1:29

The biggest problem with eating meat is that your body isn't designed to properly consume it. Nutritionally speaking, your body gets the most benefit from unprocessed plant-based foods.

If you look at creatures classified as carnivores you'll see they have certain characteristics. They have a certain physiological makeup that reflects what they are supposed to eat. A few of these are:

Claws and Sharp Front Teeth

The claws are used for killing and the big front teeth are used for tearing the flesh of their prey.

Acidic Saliva

The acids in the saliva are meant to begin digesting their raw meat immediately.

Stomach Acids More Powerful than Herbivores

Some species of carnivores have stomach acids that are up to 20 times more powerful in some cases. The food is broken down quickly in the stomach because the length of the intestines is short.

Which brings us to the next point ...

The Intestine of Carnivores is Short and Smooth

A carnivore's intestines are able to absorb the nutrients within raw meat quickly. The meat doesn't have a chance to start rotting inside the animal. The raw meat is able to move through the intestines quickly because its intestinal walls are smooth.

No Need for Fiber Inside the Intestine

Carnivores don't need fiber in their diets in order to "sweep out" food inside their digestive tract.

Ability to Handle Cholesterol

Carnivore systems have a natural ability to handle large amounts of cholesterol in their system because it's a natural byproduct of fleshy food.

Does this description of a carnivore's physiology match that of human beings? No, not at all. Also consider that when carnivores consume meat in the wild they eat the flesh raw.

One counter argument to this is that man is an "omnivore," which is a creature meant to eat both plants and animals. This is technically true to some extent, especially given the fact that there will often be tiny creatures on our garden vegetables. But for human beings to consume most meat safely it needs to be cooked.

Consuming uncooked meats is dangerous for us and carries health risks. Are you be willing to eat most meat uncooked (as omnivores in nature do)? Probably not. With this in mind, let's now look at a few characteristics of herbivores (plant eaters):

1) Flat Back Teeth (including Molars) for Chewing

2) Saliva is alkaline and not acidic. This is to help in the digestion of plant-based foods.

3) Too Much Stomach Acidity is Problematic. Think about the problem of acid-reflux in humans ... when stomach acid activity becomes overwhelming.

4) Long Length of the Intestine. This allows for a long, slow digestive process within the intestinal tract.

5) The Shape of Intestines Isn't Smooth; It's Full of Pouches. This helps the plant food to even further break down so nutrients can be absorbed into the body through the walls of the intestine.

6) Need Fiber in the Diet. The fiber acts as a broom to sweep out the plant material and keep it moving through the digestive process.

7) No Need for Cholesterol. Excess Cholesterol in the body will create problems for an herbivore.

Now, let's ask, "*Are our bodies more like herbivores or carnivores?*" Our bodies match the profile of herbivores in every way.

Here are a few more traits of herbivores that human beings have (keep in mind that carnivores do not possess these):

-- Flat Nails

-- Ability to perspire in order to regulate body temperature

-- Developed facial muscles for chewing

-- Widen jaw angle

-- The location of the jaw joint is above the molars

-- Full side-to-side and front to back jaw motion

-- Small mouth opening compared to head size

-- Broad flat back tooth shape
-- Short front canine teeth
-- Ability to chew extensively
-- Stomach acidity with a ph range between 4 and 5 when food is inside
-- Food stays in stomach for less than 30% of the total time for digestion
-- Long colon
-- Liver can't detoxify Vitamin A
-- Kidney produces urine that is mildly concentrated[18]

When you eat meat it contains no fiber at all. Its journey through your intestines is slow and sluggish. It gets caught and trapped in the pockets or your intestines and much of it begins to rot while still inside. (Have you ever seen pictures of portions of a human intestine that is gummed up with rotting fecal matter? It's not pretty).

If all the meat doesn't move through your intestines quickly it gets trapped inside the lining for an extended period of time. Then your body can begin to absorb toxins from the rotting flesh that were supposed to have been removed.

There is direct link between the consumption of animal-based food products, such as meat and dairy, with cancer. Dr. Neal Barnard writes, *"What seems to be going on is that the fatty foods - meats, dairy products, fried foods - tend to cause the hormones in a woman's or man's body to increase ... they increase when we have fattier diets, and, in turn, those hormonal surges can trigger the onset of cancer or make cancer more likely to occur."*[19]

According to recent statistics, as many as 23% of Americans will die of cancer. Could a significant amount of this disease be caused by what individuals are putting into their bodies? If your body was made to primarily consume plant-based foods then adapting a diet that matches your body's physiology would likely help prevent disease.

11

An Interview with Faye Lambeth
Testimony of Healing from Gastro-Intestinal Problems, Leg Pain and Severe Nausea

I am a teacher of music/piano at a private school in Florida. Jim, who is my husband, and I, live in the Apopka area, which is right near Orlando. We've been here almost 16 years.

I'm a native Floridian. I was born and raised here and then met Jim while we were both attending college in Tennessee. We've lived in several states but ended up coming back to Florida. We love it here.

Jim and I are parents of a son and daughter, and now we're the grandparents of 3 boys ... with another boy on the way. My husband is also a teacher and vice-principal of an elementary school here in town. We've both dedicated ourselves to teaching children.

Each year we've lived here, I've always had 4 piano recitals a year with my students. About 6 years ago, on the day of one of these recitals, I had an anxiety attack. This attack got so bad that I had to be taken to our doctor who waited for me after hours. That event turned out to be the start of a condition where doctors constantly prescribed medications for me. Over the years there were over thirty different ones.

Doctors immediately began giving me medications for the anxiety. The doctors never pinpointed why I had the attack. But it was so bad I couldn't go to the recital that night.

Soon afterwards, I started having stomach pains -- off and on. I went back to my doctor and told him about this and he prescribed more medications. None of them worked, so he suggested that I go to a Gastroenterologist to be checked out. So I followed his advice and saw a GI physician. In the meantime, I began experiencing severe bouts with nausea and acid reflux. These terrible periods of sickness lasted, off and on, for over 4 years.

Those years were filled with doctor visits and hospital stays lasting up to 4 days at a time. Different medical staffs ran multiple tests that included: MRIs, ultrasounds, and blood work. The GI doctor ran just about every test you can imagine ... sometimes twice during one hospital stay.

There were also more trips to the ER during this 4-year period. The doctors there prescribed medications also, while trying to find out if this was a digestive problem or not.

I got very anxious about my condition at times. So much so, that my medical doctor eventually suggested I go see a psychiatrist. Since I'd never been someone who experienced very much sickness during my 59 years of life up to this point, I think I was becoming very worried about my health.

Nobody seemed to be able to find out what was going on in my body. I'd always been a firm believer that if I was sick I'd go to the doctor's, get diagnosed, and then take care of things to get it over with. But with these bouts of severe sickness it wasn't happening.

I eventually did go see a psychiatrist, whom I really liked personally. He was very nice and talked with me extensively about my illness. In the end, however, all he was able to do was prescribe more medications.

I keep bringing the fact that the doctors were always prescribing medications to me because it seems all they were able to do is try various drugs for my condition for several weeks at a time. When that drug didn't work they'd try another one. And when that one didn't work they'd try something else. There were always changes in my prescriptions and I ended up being prescribed many different kinds of drugs.

My son is a physical therapist. He told me he had a patient who was a dietician who might be able to help. So I went to her and she suggested some dietary changes, which I did try. But they didn't help. It ended up being just another failed attempt to get well that went nowhere.

"Restless Legs ... and Extreme Pain"

About 4 ½ years into this period of sickness a new symptom appeared. The school where I teach has 2 large buildings. I teach in one building. But every half hour I'd have a different piano lesson, which required me to walk from one building to the next one so I could pick up the next student that I'd be teaching. So I was required to walk a lot each day.

Towards the end of 2007, as I was walking at school between the buildings, the top of my leg started hurting terribly. The pain increased so badly that I ended up having to leave school for the rest of that school year. I had to explain to the school's Principal that it hurt too bad to come in and work. I just couldn't walk. So here I was ... now having to quit work.

At this point with my illness I also began experiencing what is often called "restless legs." My legs would shake a lot and when I'd lie down it would often appear as if my legs were in motion to ride a bicycle. They were just constantly moving. I had difficulty staying in bed because I was so restless. I'd often sleep on the couch when I did sleep. I was very scared about what was going on.

I went to see more doctors once again. But they didn't have a clue as to what was wrong with me because all of my tests came back negative. They just didn't know how to treat me.

I continued to see my doctors though. On New Year's Eve I was hurting so bad in my body that I asked my husband to take me to the ER. I said, "*Something is going on in my body, but I don't know what it is.*" My daughter was here with us that night. She is a nurse and was very concerned about my extreme pain that started in my chest down to my legs.

The ER ran more tests, and also did blood work on me again. We were there several hours that night but they couldn't find the cause. So we went back home and things continued off and on. On January 23, 2008 I had to go back to the ER because of the pain in my body. Jim and I spent 7 hours there having all kind of tests run. The doctor finally came in and said, "*Faye, we don't know what's wrong with you. Every test we've run tonight has come back negative.*"

The only remedy the ER doctor offered, of course, was to write me another prescription. He also told me to see my doctors the following day. At this point, Jim and I went out to our car and talked about how the doctors had given me every prescription they could think of and yet nothing was working.

I made appointments the next day to go see both my family doctor and the Gastro-Intestinal doctor. My primary care physician said, "*Faye, I don't know what's wrong. I have no idea.*" So he wrote me another prescription. Then the GI doctor said the same thing, "*Faye, I don't know what's wrong with you. We have no answers for this.*" He then wrote me a prescription too.

Some of the prescriptions I'd been taking were for masking the symptoms of illness, such as pain and anxiety. Others were to try and help my digestive system function properly. This included problems with nausea and acid reflux. But none of the tests where showing anything wrong.

After getting another prescription from my family doctor I went out to the car and tore it up along with the ones from the ER doctor and the GI doctor. I told Jim, "*I'm through with these medicines. We must find another way.*"

By this time, my husband and I were really praying for some kind of genuine help. We didn't know what to do next.

One morning soon afterwards, Jim said to me, "*Let's go for a walk. Maybe getting out of the house a little bit will be good for you?*" So we went outside and started walking down the street and I said, "*Jim, I can't walk anymore. The strength in my legs is totally gone and they hurt very bad.*"

When I couldn't even go for a short walk with Jim down the block of our housing development I really thought I might be dying ... that my body could be shutting down. So we came back to the house, I sat down on the couch, and we prayed for direction.

Jim got on the computer and began doing some research. He was looking for some type of alternative remedy that might help, since conventional medicine wasn't working.

He called a couple of places but nothing seemed to click. A friend of mine had given me a magazine from a place called Hallelujah Acres a couple of months before this and Jim remembered that name, so he typed it into the search engine online and found their information. He ended up speaking to a wonderful couple that runs one of their "Lifestyle Centers" in North Carolina. Jim really hit it off with them and decided we should go to their health retreat for a week.

There was something about that conversation Jim had with this couple that clicked. They seemed to be very knowledgeable about digestive health problems and genuinely concerned about my condition. They made no promises whatsoever that I'd get better. But they were willing to share some very specific diet changes that I could make immediately, which targeted my severe digestive problems.

When we did finally arrive at this retreat center we began learning about the importance of 3 things: diet, exercise and getting out into the sun. These were factors Jim and I had always believed were factors in health. But we never really focused on them during my illness.

We both thought we'd been living a pretty healthy lifestyle up to that point. We were both vegetarians already. We'd quit eating meat back around 1993. But we were about to learn this wasn't enough.

Being 7th Day Adventists, we had already received some diet counseling years ago through our church affiliation. When we got to the health retreat though, I began to see how much of what we were learning about was similar to what I'd heard about through some our denomination's teachings. But these were things that Jim and I never really focused on, even though the materials had always been available to us.

They also talked a lot about the condition of our foods today, including the use of pesticides and fertilizers. Those are things that may affect health.

We arrived at the retreat on a Sunday afternoon. They pureed my food for a couple of days because of the digestive problems I'd been experiencing. Then they slowly introduced some solid foods back into my meals. Our meals consisted of plant-based foods -- 85% raw and 15% cooked -- which included lots of juicing, especially carrot juice.

We still follow this same program today. Every morning we consume about four different kinds of juices and organic supplements.

"There Was No Pain Anywhere"

For most of this trip, I was still hurting just as badly as before we'd arrived. On Thursday, we were supposed to take a ride to Shelby, North Carolina (about an hour and a half each way) to see the main headquarters for Hallelujah Acres with everyone else that was attending the health retreat that week.

I'd been up all Wednesday night feeling very sick, so I didn't know if I could go or not. I spent a lot of time sitting in the tub, trying to rub my legs because they were hurting and I was feeling miserable.

I felt as if I didn't want to go anywhere on Thursday. But I decided to get dressed and see how I felt by the time the group was getting ready to leave. So just before everyone took off for the ride I decided to go.

A little way into this daytrip I noticed something. I said to Jim, "*Look, my legs aren't moving ... they're not restless.*" When we arrived at our destination, I was able to go with the group and walk through the place. And I was also able to sit with everyone else and have lunch. Then I traveled back to the retreat center with our group without having restless legs for the entire journey.

By the time we arrived back to the retreat in the afternoon all of the pain in my body had left. The terrible pain just hadn't left my legs; there was no pain anywhere in my body.

Jim and I didn't say anything to anyone at first because there were periods before where I'd have pain, and then no pain, and then pain again. But I went to bed that night and slept well, then got up on Friday morning still feeling very good. I shared with our group that I had no restless legs and no pain in my body.

We then had breakfast that morning and went for a walk down to a waterfall. The entire walk was over a mile long. I almost couldn't believe it. I kept thinking, "*When is the pain going to start again ... when is it going to come?*" But it didn't.

We drove back to Orlando afterwards, cleaned out our pantry of all processed foods and went out and bought fresh organic foods. That has been just over a year and 2 months ago.

We're still on this diet plan. We share it with anyone who asks us about it. I truly believe now that living foods, exercise and sunshine is the way to go.

My healing was really evident just 4 days after changing my diet. That certainly isn't the case with everybody. It's a rare exception. But I'll take it!

The unhealthy foods I used to enjoy before almost seem like poison to me now. I know how sick I was and I don't want to go back. So staying with this diet hasn't been that hard for me. I truly believe this is the way we should be feeding our bodies.

Information is readily available nowadays regarding foods that are known to cause health problems. Anyone can research what is in meats today. And people can read about how the use of pesticides and fertilizer in out food supply is also widespread.

One thing I would have hated to give up after changing my diet was being able to use my local grocery store. But I can still shop there because they have aisles with organic sections in them. There are lots of organic things I can buy there. It means lots of other people are interested in eating healthy, which is great.

I've notified the 3 doctors and the dietician I'd seen pretty regularly up to this point and told them my story. They were in awe. My primary medical doctor said, "*Faye, this is the best thing for you. I think I mentioned diet to you when you were so sick.*" I replied, "*You know, you may have, but I really needed somebody to lay out a program for me, with directions on what to eat and how to prepare it. That is what really helped me.*" I was glad my primary care physician was especially encouraging regarding this.

I encourage people to check out health food stores. Go to your local grocery and see what is available with regards to organic foods. There is no reason to not try raw organic eating today.

Jim and I are both walking over 3 miles a day right now. I take no medications anymore. And we both feel great. (The leaders at the retreat center were very diligent to say that nobody should ever go off any medications whatsoever except under their own doctor's supervision. This is especially important if someone is taking medications for serious conditions, which includes insulin for diabetes and prescriptions for heart conditions).

I immediately went to my doctor and had him run some blood tests on me to make sure I was okay. And I still have him run those often.

During the course of my 4½ years of sickness, I'd gained 66 pounds. I was bloated from not eating right, not exercising, and taking all of the medications. As of today, I've lost 51 pounds. I only have a few more to lose and I'll be back to the weight I was at before getting very sick.

We live in a town where a lot of people know me and saw how sick I was. Many of them come to me and ask, "*What did you do to get better? You look so good!*" My health change is a testimony that eating this way can make a huge difference in a person's health. I'd encourage anyone to try this lifestyle. It will probably help you. If you don't like it, and it doesn't cure you, then the odds are it still won't hurt you.

Thanks to my family standing by me, my life is back to normal activities. There are so many things I was missing, like: concerts, annual family outings to the beach, not being able to hold my grandson for fear of falling with him and church activities.

I'm thankful to God for bringing us to a natural lifestyle that He gave us in the beginning.

12

An Interview with
Mariana Pina-Bergtold
Testimony of Healing from Breast Cancer

Note: *Mariana is a macrobiotic cook. Even though she would agree
with many of the concepts associated with a mostly raw vegan food diet
she isn't a proponent of a strictly raw foods diet or veganism per se.
She isn't opposed to anyone eating small amounts of organic meats or
certain kinds of fish. As you will see, however, her own physical
healing incorporated a largely organic, whole foods approach that
illustrates once again how adopting a diet that replaces harmful foods
with high-quality ones can bring dramatic healing. Her personal
testimony is part of an inspirational story that comprises an important
chapter in this book.*

I currently work as a full-time paralegal. But I'm also a
macrobiotic chef and co-owner of a vegan deli in Pittsfield,
MA called The Dancing Vegan.

I was born in northern California and orphaned when I
was 2 years old. That meant I basically became a "state"
child for the next 8 years. When I was about 9 ½ or 10
years old, I was adopted and moved to the Napa Valley. I
left home when I was very young after growing up in that
area.

When I was a young child I'd been prescribed the drugs
Ritalin and Seconal. I also had to deal with a lot of physical
problems that came from abuse. As a result, I was one of

those kids who was sick all the time. Even as a child, I spent a lot of time in the hospital.

Poor health continued to be a part of my life into my teenage and young adult years. On top of that, I started drinking alcohol and doing drugs when I was young ... until about the age of 20. Then I stopped because I nearly died. At that point in my life I was very physically sick.

"Non-Hodgkin's Lymphatic Cancer"

Whenever I got sick I did all of the things one is supposed to do: go to the doctor, take medications, get surgeries, etc. I also began eating what I thought was a healthy diet. I was always able to procure the best foods because of my work-connection to restaurants.

When I was in my 20s I was working a lot and I was under a lot of stress. At 25 years of age I experienced an ectopic (tubal) pregnancy. The doctors ended up giving me chemotherapy because of the complications that resulted. That made me very ill.

There was also a new drug study going on and I was given this new drug to try out as a patient to see if it would help me recover. The doctors, however, administered an overdose of it and my kidneys shut down. I almost died. Physicians had to put me on dialysis for a while afterwards.

I vowed that I'd never receive chemotherapy again. That was during the 1980s. Chemo drugs back then were even more draconian than they are now.

More health problems came when I entered my 30s. I had a hysterectomy, which really pushed me down a path towards health decline. And during this timeframe I changed professions and became a paralegal. That meant I had to switch gears from what I'd been doing as a chef. All of that tended to make my health even worse.

When I was around 34 or 35 there were periods when I was so sick I couldn't work at all. The pain in my body got so bad it was impossible to work. Up to that point I never connected my health problems with diet at all. I continued taking a lot of medications, including antibiotics and painkillers.

There was a point where I had to stop working for about 9 months straight. I was sick in bed most of the time and constantly going to the doctor. But I just kept getting sicker and sicker. I also started having physical maladies I'd never had before.

Constantly being in bed was totally unlike me because I didn't like spending time in bed. I was the kind of person who was always busy. There were times when I was so busy I'd only sleep a couple of hours a night.

In the fall of 2000 I went to the doctor's for a mammogram and regular physical checkup and they found a lump underneath the breast tissue. They did a biopsy and found out it was cancerous. They wanted to do a bone marrow tap and "stage" me. I did let them do that and the report came back that it was non-Hodgkin's lymphatic cancer. I thanked the doctors and then left.

It so happened that I was a part of a very ineffective health insurance plan in the Midwest at that time. I really believe that HMO ended up killing more people than it helped people get well. It was one of those in-house, all-inclusive type of health plans. They don't allow for "second" opinions or things like that. So a patient was kind of stuck if they felt like they needed more than what was offered to them within that system.

"They Wanted to Administer Chemo"

About a week after my cancer diagnosis I got into my car and drove cross-country to a place called the Kushi Institute here in Massachusetts. The Kushi Institute is a macrobiotic healing & educational center. It's in the middle of nowhere in a town called Beckett.

Kushi offers classes, including one called, "*Way to Health*," which is exceptional. They teach how to approach macrobiotic cooking, what it means and how to apply it to your life. After arriving in Massachusetts I started working at Kushi and eating the macrobiotic foods prepared there.

I'd heard about Kushi through the daughter of a friend of mine. She had come over to cook some rice for me a couple of weeks before I left for Kushi. She directed me towards this diet.

I started feeling better from the macrobiotic diet right away. It was the first time in a while that I'd been able to get out of bed, get in the shower and stay up walking around for 6 hours at a time. It was amazing. This started happening after just 5 or 6 days of being on a macrobiotic diet.

I went to Kushi because I knew I couldn't go through what the doctors who'd diagnosed me were going to prescribe. They wanted to administer surgery, chemo, radiation, a bone marrow transplant and all of that insanity. I knew it would kill me. So I turned my back on it and walked away.

When I got to Kushi I started working there as a volunteer in housekeeping. I kind of worked my way up from there and stayed for about a year and a half. Then I moved to Pittsfield, which is a town nearby.

After moving here I started practicing macrobiotics myself with the help of a woman who became my mentor. (Having a mentor can be very helpful for anyone who is approaching macrobiotics if they're sick).

I went to work for a lawyer here in town. He took me on even while I was still sick and he has been very good to me. This gentleman even allowed me to work from home when I couldn't come in at times because I was too sick to come into the office.

This allowed me to continue learning how to eat healthy and construct a healthy lifestyle for myself. That was very big. When you try and work 20 hours a day, like I'd done in years past, it won't work. We all have to learn how to do things and live in such a way that we work with the time clock each of us have in our body.

I've also discovered that if I'm depressed it can have a lot to do with what is going on in my system. There are certain areas of our body that need to be balanced with proper nutrition. I needed to take responsibility for what I was doing with my body when it came to food.

"Natural Healing"

Taking control of what we put into our mouths can be hard because few of us want to take responsibility for what we're eating. If we eat something just because we like the way it tastes then consuming a proper diet will be a real battle.

When I came into macrobiotics it took me a few years to get to the place where the only meat I was eating was fish. I didn't eat much meat, but once in a while I did. Then I went to just eating fish, but started getting sick from even that because there are so many chemicals in it. So I eliminated fish from my diet also.

So as you can see, I started out in macrobiotics, which is not necessarily vegan. I'm now basically vegan in my own diet, but I don't discount the possibility of adjusting the foods I may eat in the future, depending upon my health. More than anything, my health would dictate any diet changes I might make.

When I finally eliminated fish from my diet then I virtually became a vegan by definition. When I started the restaurant I wanted to make it vegan, but also include macrobiotic and vegetarian elements within it.

One concept behind macrobiotic food preparation is that you first try to gather foods from your regional and seasonal zone. Then you try to match those foods with what your own body needs. Since we're all individuals we all have individual nutritional needs.

Each of our bodies will react to different foods in different ways. If you become in tune with your body then you can find out what it needs. I eat more beans and greens than grains. This is important for me because I feel more comfortable when I eat more beans. My body seems to be really happy when I do this. So it's about learning what your body needs and how it responds to certain things.

The quality of most food here in the U.S. today isn't very good. I really believe a lot of people are ill today just based upon food quality. People get sick with diseases they really shouldn't be getting. It's the food that is killing them.

After making the switch to a healthy macrobiotic diet one of the first things I noticed was that I was getting my energy back. But one big thing I had to deal with was the fact I'd gained around 140 pounds of extra weight during my years of sickness. My lymphatic system was shot.

I can totally empathize with anyone who has a weight problem. I was in so much misery from that weight. My back, legs and knees constantly hurt. I had no mobility. But as I got better the weight came off. It didn't come off right away. A lot of people will come to macrobiotics and start dropping weight immediately. But I was not that person.

It took me 3 years to finally lose all of that extra weight. I initially lost around 40 pounds and then the rest of it came off slowly. It was so great not to have my back and legs always hurting.

There had been a point in my life where I'd had 15 surgeries in 12 years. There was a lot of nerve damage in my body because of all the cutting I endured. It was a big deal for me to finally "get my body back."

Walking or standing for any length of time started to be a problem for me when I was only in my 30s. I was also diagnosed with fibromyalgia at that time. I can tell you I don't have problems associated with those things anymore. It took me a long time to get rid of them. But they did finally go away.

Nothing good that happened to me happened overnight. A lot of people come into a natural diet and think that in just 6 months they can be cured. But natural healing can take a 5-7 year span of time. It can take a few years for your body to really change.

I've got pictures of myself when I first came to Kushi and if you compare them with today it's as if I'm a whole different person. To see that transformation is really amazing.

"Feeling Lighter"

When I first started changing my diet I changed about 80% of it right away. But I was not able to let go of certain things immediately. I was a horrible sugar junkie. I ate sugar constantly and had terrible pancreatic problems as a result. That sugar was usually in the form of hard candy or chocolate. Those kinds of addictions started changing gradually through my new food.

If I go crazy for a food nowadays I may, for example, eat 20 olives because I've got a temporary salt craving. The cravings in my body are much more centered now. When I was on medications all the time, the sugar, orange juice and meat I'd consumed really affected the balance of my body.

The biggest single change I made immediately was going organic. I can honestly say that eating organic alone (and I can now attest to this from years of eating this way) probably affects my health by as much as 60%. If I go out and eat in a Chinese restaurant then I'm sick for the next 3 days. That is about food quality. What is in the food? It's amazing how much people don't realize what they're eating.

For me, the hardest part about changing my diet was feeling "lighter." I know that sounds weird, but when you don't eat meat or dairy you feel light inside. Your body feels lighter. Your stomach feels lighter. It's not that you feel "hungry," you just feel "lighter." The last time I had a steak I remember thinking, *"Oh, how am I going to move?"* But I do not feel that way now.

If somebody were considering a diet change I'd tell him or her the single most important thing is to eat organically. The second biggest thing would be getting off the sugar. And the third biggest thing would be to get off animal products. Start eating more beans. Get off dairy.

If you feel like you have to eat meat then consume very light fish. Try to do that. But as much as you can, get yourself away from processed foods and move towards organic whole foods.

"Try Eating Organic for a Week"

What is the status of my health right now? I think this is probably the first winter since I've lived here that I haven't had any pneumonia or bronchitis. My health is pretty good right now. I could work 14 hours at the restaurant if I needed to. And I can put in as many hours as I need to at the law firm. Do I have days where I feel "achy" occasionally? Yes. But the reality of things is my health is very good.

If anyone is skeptical that simply changing their diet can bring healing from serious health issues I'd tell them to try eating organic for a week. If they want to still eat meat and all of that then they can. But don't eat anything unless it's organic. If they'd just go organic I'd think they'd notice differences in their body and find that the taste of their food would be amazing. And I think they'd feel better too.

The organic difference is big. I really feel like this is where we've fallen off the wagon in our world. When we started trying to preserve foods for longer than nature intended for them to be preserved then that was a major

109

error. Compromising the food in such a way compromises our health.

There is a great book out there called, *"The Hip Chicks Guide to Macrobiotics,"* by Jessica Porter. It's a great book because she sort of modernized macrobiotics for people today. One thing you have to realize about macrobiotics is that it changes. What was done 30 years ago is different than what is recommended today because it tries to account for changes that take place within our current supply of natural foods. Jessica's book is a very easy read and most of the recipes are very light.

Another resource would be a woman who does a series on PBS. Her name is Christina Pirello and she is amazing. She is a whole foods macrobiotic chef and she has written quite a few books, including one called, *"Cooking the Whole Foods Way."*

If you're trying to switch to a macrobiotics diet, or whole foods diet, or vegan diet then vegan restaurants can really come in handy (although a lot of vegan restaurants use sugar, which their clientele might or might not know). These restaurants generally have a better quality of food though. The food is often organic and specially prepared too.

If you visit vegan restaurants then you can experience a cross section of new tastes. You'll also get to experience new vegetables used in new situations (from your standpoint) with grains and beans. You'll also be exposed to new varieties of foods you didn't know about because you're not going to make yourself 5 or 6 different kinds of dishes for every mealtime at home.

You don't want to get bored with your food. If you do then you're not going to want to change your diet and eat healthy. So I encourage people to go out and try and find whole foods markets and co-ops and places like that.

I also suggest they go out and enjoy good foods already prepared at vegan restaurants. Utilize these kinds of places

110

when trying to change your diet. Getting out and experiencing new foods that have been prepared in a healthy way is very big!

You should also begin experiencing some vegan treats. That is what happened to me. I have a job where I have to go out into the world and work. I even have to go out for lunch during the week sometimes. So I started utilizing local whole foods and vegan places and meeting new people there. I made trips to the local health food store. I started gearing my life towards those kinds of markets.

I made visiting those sorts of places a new adventure. Every time I had to travel to a new city or visit a new state I'd look up the whole foods places before my trip and then go find them. It's really fun to do things like that. I've been able to visit a lot of vegan restaurants across the country by doing this.

You'll get ideas for recipes and start tasting new things and new textures when you venture out. Over time, it'll infiltrate itself into your Standard American Diet and help change the way you eat.

"You Need Support"

I know a lot of macrobiotic chefs that do raw foods now. I think it adds to the need to lighten dishes up more. I think these foods are important, especially for many who are transitioning from having a heavy meat and dairy background.

I eat a lot of salads in the summer but not many in the winter because it's cold outside and salads tend to cool off my body. When I lived in California last year for a while I ate lots of salads and raw foods. The temperature in the area I lived was often over 100 degrees. So I ate a lot of raw foods while there.

In my opinion, raw foods are particularly important for those who're coming from a heavy meat or dairy background. That is one thing macrobiotics teaches ... the idea to be open to other things.

You need to investigate and ask questions for yourself. Try and see if something will work for you. I believe that coming off meats and dairy, processed foods and conventionally grown vegetables and fruits are the most important thing.

If you need to change your diet and "go it alone" then do it. I've seen so many people try and change to a healthy diet but their friends and family talk them out of it.

If you start eating whole foods and you drop a lot of weight, or your body reacts strangely to the new healthy food, and your friends and family try and talk you out of it, then you'll have to resolve to do it by yourself. Even though they may be well intentioned, your friends and family may end up killing you.

You need support when changing your diet. Find somebody else who is doing what you want to do and has experienced what you're experiencing and look to them for support. Having somebody that has more experience than you have in this area to guide you can make a huge difference when trying to reach your health goals.

The idea for my restaurant was borne out of my own desire to be able to go to someplace locally and get something healthy to eat. There was nothing close to where I work that fit my needs.

I really wanted to have a little café or deli that took care of local macrobiotic, kosher and vegan eaters. I also wanted to offer a local bakery that didn't use sugar. We use just rice syrup, maple sugar and agave for sweeteners. I wanted to show people that you could have good tasting things without using sugar or dairy products.

The reason I opened the Dancing Vegan in Pittsfield, MA is because there was a need for an organic vegan restaurant in the Berkshires to accommodate the many cultural and ethnic groups residing and visiting. I am happy

112

that I am able to begin to fill that void and hope others will join me.

I've got people coming into the restaurant everyday and telling me they're getting sick and they've heard they should try this stuff. Now I get to see big, 300-pound guys go out the door eating vegan lasagna and loving it. Then they come back and ask for vegan cookies that don't have any sugar in them because they like the way they taste. It's wonderful!

....

Mariana Pina-Bergtold's vegan deli, the Dancing Vegan, is located in Pittsfield, Massachusetts. More information about Mariana's vegan fares and treats can be found on the DancingVegan's website:
http://www.thedancingvegan.com
An online article featuring Mariana's deli is at:
http://www.berkshireeagle.com/ci_11624008?source=most_emailed

13
Dead Food Versus Living Food

What does the phrase, "Dead Foods" refer to in our reference to diet? From the perspective of raw living foods, dead foods are ones that have been processed in such a way that their natural living enzymes and composition has been altered (often to preserve shelf life). An example of "dead" foods is anything that comes out of can, box or sealed package considered edible for weeks or months.

Most foods are "processed" in a way that strips them of their natural enzymes, vitamins and nutrients. They can also end up filling your body with unhealthy chemicals and carcinogenic materials. The amount of chemicals and artificial additives used in foods today is staggering.

The terrible truth is that when you're in the supermarket, every aisle apart from the produce section is filled with "dead" products. Most processed foods are stripped of vital vitamins and nutrients and then reconstituted in such a way that shelf life is enhanced. Then they're loaded with sugar and artificial flavors in order to make them "tasty" for paying consumers.

Any foodstuff offered for sale that comes in a can, box, jar, or sealed bag is potentially harmful to your system. They've either been heated (before freezing or other processing) or stripped completely of most of their nutrients. With the all-natural life-giving properties of these products removed they're nutritionally very poor. This reality has created a Western culture that is largely over-fed yet under-nourished.

Many people are completely surprised to discover that processed foods such as white rice, pasta and white breads are also void of nutrition. When rice is "refined" in the way white rice is processed its kernels are stripped of the minerals, fiber, phytochemicals and vitamins present at harvest (the good, nutritious stuff). Then it's packaged for consumption.

Other Harmful Food Products

The following is a list of other popular food products that can destroy health. The health problems caused by these products are widely known and well documented.

White Sugar: Refined sugar is a leading cause of health problems today. At the beginning of the 20th century the average American only ingested about 5 pounds of it per year. Today, that amount has exploded to an average of 170 pounds a year – per person! That amounts to over 50 teaspoons of sugar per day. A single can of soda, for example, contains nearly 11 teaspoons of sugar. It can be found in cereals, ice cream and packaged food products.

Sugar suppresses your body's immune system, contains empty calories (void of nutrition) and can lead to conditions such as obesity, diabetes, ADD, cancer and depression, just to name a few.

White Salt: Our bodies only require a very small amount of sodium chloride (salt). This small amount can easily be obtained in a raw vegetable such as celery. Most Americans ingest far too much, however, in foods such as breakfast cereals, hot dogs, commercial salad dressings, deli meats, canned goods and processed cheese.

Too much salt contributes to a variety of health problems, including: arterial sclerosis, kidney stones, hypertension, liver dysfunction and high blood pressure.

White Flour: This dead food is nutritionally worthless. To create white flour a producer has to take natural grains of wheat and strip them of their bran and wheat germ. What is leftover is then ground up into a power and bleached.

The resulting substance contains no fiber and no living enzymes. It can gum up your system and lead to constipation. It can also coat the walls of your intestine and prevent vital nutrients in living foods from passing into your system during the digestive process.

Caffeine: This is the drug of choice for many individuals. This substance is found in coffee, chocolate and certain sodas and teas.

Caffeine is highly addictive (just try going off coffee if you drink it regularly) and toxic to the body. It constricts blood vessels and makes the heart beat faster. This causes that rush of adrenalin most individuals enjoy when drinking their coffee. Caffeine can contribute to high blood pressure, kidney damage, liver damage, heart attacks, stroke and osteoporosis.

Dead Meat

Dr. T. Colin Campbell, who authored *The China Study*, concluded that ingesting even small amounts of animal products significantly increases your chances for degenerative diseases, especially cancer.

In one study, Dr. Campbell describes an experiment where he introduced cancer inside an animal. He was able to keep the cancer from spreading by feeding the animal a vegan diet. But the cancer started to grow rapidly after he added cow's milk into the animal's diet.[20]

Meat may also be considered to be a "dead" food apart from the fact that most meats aren't consumed in raw form. Most meats are processed in such a way that fills them with artificial substances.

Take cattle for instance. Being raised prior to slaughter includes use of hormones designed to stimulate growth and add fat. Howard Lyman's book, *Mad Cowboy* is an insider's look into the modern meat producing cattle industry. Reading it will make you look at meat production in a whole new light.

Before the advent of the widespread use of chemicals in the 20th century, beef would typically contain 3-5% fat. Today's cattle contain anywhere between 20-40% of fat. The same is true of pork and chicken.

When you eat meat it's possible to ingest up to 100 pounds of fat into your system during the course of a year. On top of that, you're ingesting a host of unwanted chemicals and hormones into your body. It's not exactly the stuff I'd want to be eating if I were trying to get rid of cancer.

"What about protein?" many are quick to ask. *"Don't I need to eat meat in order to obtain protein?"* The answer is simply, "*No.*" There is only 5.4 grams of protein in 100 calories of steak, but 11.2 grams in 100 calories of broccoli. Romaine lettuce has even more -- 11.6 grams.

Think about huge vegetarian animals, like cows, gorillas, hippopotamuses and elephants. Where did they consume the protein necessary to grow so big? The point here is that you can get all of the protein you need from plant food. You don't need to eat any disease-causing meats in order to feed your body adequate amounts of protein.

Meat also creates excess uric acid in the body. Uric acid is a chemical produced by the body to break down certain substances produced by certain foods. As Dr. Rowen Pfeifer has noted, *"Your body can process the uric acid of only a very small amount of meat every day - about 4 ounces. When you're taking in anywhere from 8 to 25 ounces of meat a day, you've got all this uric acid your body cannot eliminate. Then it crystallizes. It's like broken glass. And it tends to settle in your joints, actually shredding the cartilage."*[21]

Before I met my wife her family had changed their diet for about 2 years in order to try and help my soon-to-be bride get better from a neurological condition she suffered with at the time. While their diet change wasn't "meat free," it did include the elimination of regular market meats that contained hormones. Her family also eliminated most products containing processed sugar, artificial ingredients and dairy.

The results were astounding. Everyone in her family lost a great deal of weight without "dieting" or counting calories in any way. My wife's nutritionist had even predicted this could happen because most commercial foods are filled with more sugars and chemicals than most people can imagine.

I remember being absolutely amazed when seeing her before-diet and after-diet pictures. The amount of artificial ingredients, including chemicals and taste enhancers in most commercial foods is unknown to most of us because they're invisible. But those things all accumulate in the body.

This means foods that are dangerous to your health don't simply include meat, but anything that comes from, or is made with, something that comes from an animal. This includes eggs, milk, cheese and other dairy products.

Most Americans consider dairy an important part of their diet because of a need for calcium. This view has been propagated and reinforced over many years by advertising from dairy producers.

The real truth, however, is that consuming dairy products can actually deplete your body of necessary calcium. Does this surprise you?

Consider the fact that Americans are among the highest consumers of dairy products in the world, yet suffer far more hip fractures than populations with much lower dairy consumption. New Guineans, for example, consume 32 times less milk than Americans, but Americans suffer 47 times more hip fractures.[22]

Consuming dairy products actually causes your body to excrete more calcium than it takes in. In other words, your body will pass more calcium out of your body through stool and urine excretions than will be absorbed into your body through the digestion process. Over time, that calcium depletion results in bone loss.

In the opinion of some researchers, the bone loss Americans suffer from consuming dairy products is a major reason why Americans (and other high dairy consuming populations) suffer more from hip fractures. Most Americans don't know that raw and whole foods, including green vegetables, sesame seeds, beans -- and even fruits such as oranges -- contain calcium that the body can use without the negative side effect triggering calcium elimination from the body.

What are Living Foods?

Living foods are largely unprocessed natural and whole foods that contain a substantially high level of living enzymes and vitamins. In the purest sense, the best living foods are organic, raw vegetables and fruits that haven't been cooked or artificially processed. Their natural enzymes haven't been "killed." Nor has their natural physical composition been changed or altered.

The best illustration I can offer is to suggest that you take a fresh carrot and cut the end off and stick it in water. After a day or two, the cut end will start growing in the water because the cells in that area are still active and alive.

If you take that same carrot, however, and heat it over 107 degrees then it will become "cooked" enough so that its living cells die. At this point, its physical properties are altered, and its benefits as a vitamin-rich food are significantly decreased because the living enzymes are no longer present.

Uncooked plant food, including fruits, vegetables, seeds and nuts contain vitamins and nutrients in their natural state. It's impossible to consume foods that are superior in nutrient quality than vegetables and fruits BEFORE they're either cooked or artificially processed to enhance shelf life.

Cooking or typical processing changes the state of natural products and makes them inferior with regards to nutritional benefit. This means the typical western diet -- which all too frequently contains few portions of uncooked fruits and vegetables, seeds or nuts -- offers a very low level of nutritional quality.

What is truly amazing isn't the fact that human beings suffer from eating foods that are so nutrient deficient. What's amazing is that the human body is able to seemingly get along well for so long without consuming foods that contain the highest degree of fresh vitamins, minerals, nutrients and fiber.

Eating is a part of the mechanics whereby your body derives life force taken from a plant's photosynthesis activity and benefits from it. Plants feed your body in a way that allows it to draw energy from the sun and nutrients from the ground as efficiently as possible. Any food that is of any benefit to your body whatsoever is attached to this process.

This means those of us with access to fresh vegetables and fruits must ask ourselves the following:

"Why eat mostly foods that are processed in such a way that their life-sustaining properties have been significantly decreased or even completely stripped away?"

"Why eat so-called "foods" that are not only deficient in vitamins and minerals (due to the way they've been processed) but are potentially toxic or even carcinogenic to the body?"

It makes no sense.

Cooked and processed foods offer less nutritional value to your body. The living enzymes are "killed," and the vitamin content is substantially reduced.

Somewhere just above 107 degrees in cooking the enzymes within organic organisms (plant or animal) start to die. At 122 degrees the food is completely dead. If cooked even more, the molecular structure of the organism becomes altered.

Man is the only creature that "cooks" food. Carnivores in nature do not cook their food. Carnivore-predator creatures in the wild consume their food "raw."

During the 1930s, Dr. Francis Pottenger conducted an experiment with 900 cats. He fed them all identically the same food, except that half of the cats ate their food raw and the other half ate it cooked. The cats eating raw food during this 9-year period suffered very little physical breakdown. But the cats that ate the cooked food began to suffer the same kinds of chronic disease that afflict human beings in western civilization.[23]

Another story along this line comes from the 1920s. A few zookeepers tried to save money by feeding their carnivorous animals leftover cooked food, which had been obtained from local restaurants. They soon stopped the practice though because the animals started to get very sick. Some died.[24]

When modern processed foods began to become a staple in Western diets the onset of many of the chronic diseases we face today became more common. Even though we're living longer, and have access to greater amounts and more varieties of food than ever before, diseases such as cancer are now commonplace.

Cancer used to be a disease that mainly afflicted "old" people. But more and more cancers began appearing in younger generations after the advent of modern food production. Did you know that today, after accidents, cancer is the number one killer disease of children?

According to the *National Center for Health Statistics*, the leading causes of death among all members of the US population in 2005 were:

Heart disease: 652,091
Cancer: 559,312

121

Stroke (cerebrovascular diseases): 143,579
Chronic lower respiratory diseases: 130,933
Accidents (unintentional injuries): 117,809
Diabetes: 75,119
Alzheimer's disease: 71,599
Influenza/Pneumonia: 63,001
Nephritis, nephrotic syndrome, and nephrosis: 43,901
Septicemia: 34,136

Eating a living plant-based diet simply means consuming as many vegetables and fruits in their natural, raw, uncooked condition that you can. That is the point their nutritional value is of the highest value to your body.

It stands to reason that a diet of living foods should not only help prevent many diseases, but actually bring about remission in a large number of them if wrong diet was a primary trigger for their onset to begin with. There are many testimonies from individuals once stricken with these kinds of diseases (and now well) that bear out this theory.

One thing to consider is that simply eating and feeling "full" doesn't mean your body is getting the vitamins and nutrients it needs to be healthy. It's possible to be "overweight," yet "undernourished." This is what is going on in Western culture today.

When you eat a healthy plant-based diet then you may very well discover not only good health but also that you can eat as much as you want and your body will move towards an ideal weight. In other words, you won't have to "go on a diet" because you're consuming a proper diet.

This brings us to another issue. Is cooked food ever okay? At the risk of sounding contradictory to what I've just written, I'm going to say, "*Yes.*"

While eating organic, raw, living plant food is ideal, the actual practice of going "totally raw" in one's diet can be overwhelming for many individuals. So in the interest of trying to implement as much of a raw diet as possible a large number of individuals have discovered they can still enjoy stellar health results while consuming a small percentage of cooked vegetables (and other plant-based foods).

In other words, eating a small percentage of cooked plant food has helped many raw food enthusiasts adhere to a 99.9% plant-based diet. And that seems to be much more important for gaining health than fretting over whether or not a low percentage of cooked vegetables is also being consumed.

So if you've always enjoyed cooked foods your whole life then it may do your soul well to regularly steam, bake or roast vegetables, cook vegetable soups for dinner or serve yourself healthy portions of cooked brown rice or beans. The best part is you can still experience great health results even though a small amount of the vegetables you consume are cooked.

Why Eating "Raw" Can Enable Healing

Our bodies are composed of living cells. The vitamins and minerals consumed through our diet are necessary for both healthy cell creation and ongoing function.

Every day your human body is alive on this earth it replaces about 300 million dying cells with new ones. So the body is constantly in a state of replenishing itself in an effort to build itself back up. The theory behind eating raw foods is simple; living foods offer the highest quality materials to feed and fuel the creation and work of living cells.

As stated earlier, when you look at creatures in nature you find that each and every one of them consumes their food in a raw, natural state. Even carnivores, which are creatures that hunt other creatures, consume their food raw.

The food chain is such that creatures consume living cells in various forms. At the basis of the entire food chain is vegetation. All creatures consume either vegetation … or other creatures that have first consumed vegetation. Predators that eat other creatures do not cook their food before consuming it. They eat the flesh before it putrefies and becomes rancid.

When you cook food its cells are no longer "living." The living enzymes within the food are killed. The amount of vitamins and minerals found within food in its natural state is significantly diminished. So while it is possible to obtain vitamins and minerals in cooked foods, the process of heating up food diminishes its value to your body as a food product. In other words, if you want to get the most out of your food, you should cook as little of it as possible.

The main goal of healthy eating is to feed your body what it needs to replace dying cells with healthy cells. But if you feed your body with foods that are actually toxic to it then your body's cells can get to a point where they're being replaced with inferior quality cells ... resulting in a state of degeneration. This condition often results in many of the diseases so common today.

Most people need reading glasses starting at some point in young adulthood. I've read many testimonies from individuals now in middle age whose eyes became stronger when they switched to a living foods diet. They had to either get weaker prescription glasses or got rid of them altogether. This is just one of the many benefits that may be enjoyed by consuming a raw plant-based diet composed of living foods.

Switching from mostly dead foods to living foods allows your body to rebuild and heal itself. And this is the fundamental understanding behind the connection of diet and disease. Unhealthy diets lead to disease and a host of other physical ailments. It's not hard to find cases where debilitating and life-threatening diseases have simply gone away when the sick persons switched to a living foods diet.

Imagine ... a cure for most diseases that doesn't involve spending a fortune on costly medical procedures.

If, for example, you could choose a remedy for cancer that restored health without requiring poisonous drugs, toxic radiation or expensive surgery, would you embrace it?

You see your own body's healing ability at work whenever you get a cut on your leg, arm or finger. At first, the cut produces some blood. But your body sends messages to the cells in the area of the cut and they begin a process of coagulating the blood until it covers over the damaged skin area and forms a scab. Eventually the wounded area heals altogether as the damaged skin cells are replaced with new ones.

In the same way, your body will also try to heal itself whenever there is a problem internally. Those same self-healing properties you see on the outside are on the inside of your body too. Under the right conditions, your own body's immune system can function to get rid of cancer because it has already dealt with cancer cells successfully in the past. A person's body will normally want to fight any cancer cells that begin forming within it.

Fortunes are spent on drugs today in an effort to get rid of many ailments that would simply go away with a change in diet. The proper foundation to a healthy immune system is healthy, living cells that are fed with mostly raw living foods. Living food offers your body essential vitamins and nutrients for rebuilding damaged areas.

Can you imagine willfully damaging the internal organs of your body on any given day? Of course not! But may I suggest to you that is exactly what is happening when you eat meats and other commercially processed foods. You're potentially damaging your body and inviting diseases like cancer to take root inside you by eating the wrong foods.

Most of us also pass unhealthy eating habits off on our children. Most parents wouldn't allow little children to smoke or consume alcohol at the kitchen table. But they're happy to let them consume cookies, doughnuts, cup cakes, ice cream and candy on an almost daily basis. Those foods are socially acceptable but widely known to cause health problems.

Toxic food is harmful to the body. Ingesting foods that damage your body invites sickness. But feeding yourself living foods will help your body heal itself. In other words, living food can indirectly yet powerfully foster health in your body.

The Importance of Juicing

An important part of the living food diet recommended within this book includes drinking fresh-squeezed vegetable juices. A small amount of fruit juices are acceptable also. But unprocessed raw vegetable juices offer a valuable nutritional benefit to the body. By unprocessed, I'm referring to juice you prepare yourself using fresh vegetables, not juices found in a can, bottle or otherwise prepared through some commercial pre-packaging process.

Drinking a healthy amount of raw vegetable juice offers exceptional building material to your system as it works to replenish dying cells with new living cells. A stronger, healthier body results.

If you nourish your body with living vegetables and fruits, including juices extracted from them on a daily basis, then you'll be feeding your body the highest quality materials for building a healthy system.

The importance of juicing cannot be overstated. In order to offer your body the highest concentration of living enzymes, vitamins and nutrients you should juice. Juicing is the process by which you can extract vegetable (and fruit) juices from raw foods. If eating raw living food is important (and it is) then juicing comes on its heels.

There are a couple of reasons for juicing. First, juicing enables your body to absorb nutrients in the most direct way. Our bodies do need the fiber contained in raw foods to be fed properly. But juicing is an important supplement to eating.

There is an ongoing discussion today about whether or not vegetables and fruits nowadays contain less nutrients than they did in the early 20th century. I don't know which argument is true. But I do know the chemicals frequently used in modern food production have adversely affected much of the soil used in agriculture today. This is one reason why many raw food advocates consider organic foods superior.

Another reason to make juicing a part of your daily routine is that it's often difficult for the digestive system to process and absorb all of the nutrients within solid foods. When extracted juices are separated from the solid fibers your body can absorb the vitamins and nutrients more directly.

The juices to focus on are vegetable juices. Fruit juices should only be consumed in very limited quantities. Carrot juice has become a popular (and very successfully used) base for juicing. You could drink 100% raw carrot juice or use raw carrot juice with other vegetables in combination. For example, 70% carrot juice and 30% celery juice. Or 60% carrot juice, 20% celery juice and 20% of some other green leafy vegetable. (More information and resources for juicing are available at LivingFoodCures.com).

There are many combinations of vegetables that would work well together. Dr. Norman Walker is regarded in many circles as a pioneer of modern juicing. He spent years investigating various combinations and documented his research, including recipes, in the book, "*Fresh Vegetable and Fruit Juices.*"

Dr. Walker is a perfect example of how health benefits can be derived from juicing. He was cured of a very serious illness when in his early fifties. He became a raw food advocate and extensively juiced mostly fresh vegetable juices for the rest of his life. He lived a healthy, active life until he died in his sleep at 99 years of age.

Also consider how many Americans have been entertained watching Jay Kordich talk about juicing vegetables and fruits on television? Do you remember seeing him as "The Juiceman" on infomercials during the 1990s?

As Jay's story goes, he was 25 years old in 1948 and diagnosed with bladder cancer. The doctor said he had a golf-ball sized tumor. In his search to get well Jay became a patient of the famous physician Dr. Max Gerson, who taught Jay about juicing vegetables in order to detoxify his body and rebuild his immune system. Three months later, Jay was cancer-free.

As you can see, there are powerful health benefits to juicing vegetables. I recommend it because so many others have experienced successful results by doing it.

Vegetables should be thoroughly washed before extracting the juice. To save a bit on produce costs you might consider buying vegetables in bulk. You may also want to get a little refrigerator and reserve it just for your vegetables so you have plenty of room to store them for use throughout the week. That makes it easier to rotate them and keep track of which ones need to be used first before going bad.

It's best to drink fresh juices soon after extraction to keep the nutrients from being depleted over time. If you do all of your extracting in the morning then you can save an afternoon's juice drink inside a tight jar or container until you're ready to consume it.

It's better to drink 6-8 ounces of juice several times a day in order for your body to get the most benefit. If you're healthy then you can juice 2-3 times a day to maintain your health. But when you're fighting disease you may juice up to 6-7 times throughout the day ... an hour before and after meals.

14

An Interview with Danny Garris
Testimony of Healing from Severe Arthritis

I'm an electronics technician in North Carolina and am extremely busy running my own business. My business offers TV repair and servicing for electronics.

In 2001 I started having symptoms with arthritis. I really didn't know what it was at the time. I started having pain in my joints, along with muscle stiffness. Then I started waking up in the morning and feeling very stiff. I'd take long showers just to feel good enough to get moving in the morning.

Then I gradually began having problems even raising my arms above my head. My movement became more and more limited. Stretching became difficult and it felt like somebody was pouring concrete throughout my body. If I stood in one place for a long time, stayed on the couch for a couple of hours watching a movie, or slept for 6 hours and then tried to move, my body would be extremely stiff.

The arthritis got so bad there were mornings when I literally couldn't get out of bed. I'd just lie there for a while and then roll myself onto the floor. My joints would pop and snap. Then I'd crawl to the shower and get under the hot water for about an hour until the heat made my joints feel good enough to where I could go to work.

When things got really bad I could only work about 2 hours a day. I'd go into work as late as 12 pm ... then 1 pm ... and then as late as 2 pm on some afternoons. I'd work as best I could, then go back home and crawl into bed, starting the whole process over again.

I required more and more sleep in the mornings because I couldn't sleep at night. I also started having extreme body odor under both of my armpits. I noticed this, of course, but even if I swam in a river all day long I could get out of the water and still smell that odor. I just didn't understand what was going on.

"You'll Be in a Wheelchair Soon"

To try and find out what was the matter I began visiting all kinds of medical doctors. I had an MRI done and blood work. Eventually, I ended up spending thousands of dollars on conventional medicine through health insurance.

One medical doctor simply offered me some prescriptions when I went to see him. I asked him why he was giving them to me. I said, "*You haven't even done anything to me yet, like take an x-ray or ask any questions.*" This man was a top rheumatologist in my city. So then I asked him if he knew what was wrong with me. He replied, "*No ... try these prescriptions for 3 months and then come back to see me. If they don't work we'll try something else.*"

I did eventually have some x-rays done. They didn't show much except the fact there was inflammation throughout my body. The doctor couldn't give me any definite answers. But he did know I was suffering from some sort of autoimmune attack, although he didn't know what was causing it. This was typical of the many arthritis patients he'd seen and he said it would probably continue to get worse over time.

My blood tests showed I had very high cholesterol and very high triglycerides. I know now these things come from what you eat, but at that point I didn't know this. My uric acid levels were also very high. Today, I can look at a blood test and read it almost as good as my own doctor because the food connection makes sense to me.

When you know what the cause of something is then you can also know if you can do anything about it. The doctors were unable to really help me because they were trying to treat the symptoms and not the cause!

Things came to a point where I began searching on my own for what was wrong with my body. I spent about 2 years diligently searching, which included reading lots of books and asking my family doctor to professionally refer me to Duke University Medical Center for help. The best arthritis doctors in the world are supposedly at Duke. It took 6 months to get an appointment there, but I was able to get booked with one of the top rheumatologists in the world.

During this whole process my father began thinking something was poisoning me. People who knew me were very worried. My family doctor even said, "*At the rate you're going, you'll be in a wheelchair soon.*" My stiffness and pain was rapidly getting so bad I was no longer able to raise my arms above my shoulders and couldn't bend down. If I dropped my screwdriver and a customer was in my shop I'd have to ask the customer to bend down and pick it up.

That franticly spurred me on even more to search for some help. I began to read, read, read and read. I bought book after book on topics such as fibromyalgia and arthritis. After the symptoms became worse it became clear this wasn't just fibromyalgia. There was something else going on inside me.

"She Said There Was No Cure For It"

A couple of the books I read were, "*I Cured My Arthritis, You Can Too,*" by Margie Garrison and "*How to Eat Away Arthritis*" by Laurie M. Aesoph. Those authors really opened my eyes up to the influence of food upon this disease. In other words, people who had arthritis could try to begin eliminating certain foods in order to achieve beneficial results. I tried many of their recommendations. Even though I never achieved a complete fix, I did benefit from a lot of what I learned.

This is where I began to get the knowledge my problem may be coming from something as simple as what I was putting into my own mouth. Some of the books I read referred to fasting for a few days. So I tried it. The first fast I did incorporated honey and lemon juice mixed into my drinking water. I had no results with that. But about a month later I tried another fast that had been recommended in one of the books. I had nothing to eat for 5 days and didn't drink anything but pure distilled water. The results were amazing.

My pain had been so bad on certain days that I couldn't even get out of my car without help. The pain, muscle stiffness and swelling in my joints made it so that I had to walk inch-by-inch to get around. I couldn't even reach up to pull the chain on my ceiling fan anymore.

I'd been taking Pregnezone, and that drug caused my body to pack on weight. I weighed about 215 pounds at the start of my fast. I thought, if nothing else, doing this fast would help me lose some of that weight. But by the 4th day of this fast, about 95% of the arthritis pain in my body was gone. On the 5th day, I was bending down and raising my arms up over my head for the first time in many months.

My employees came into my shop the next day and saw me working and couldn't believe I was able to do what I was doing. They asked me what was going on because they knew how sick I'd been. When I jumped up after bending down and lifted my arms above my head they were amazed.

They knew I was fasting but didn't understand what I was learning about food. I told them that I finally had begun to learn that my (SAD) Standard American Diet was causing my poor health. And that many years of a poor unhealthy diet and lifestyle are the primary cause of up to 90% of health problems in this country. I discovered this before I went to my appointment at Duke University. This new knowledge helped me to discover that the answers and power to my own healing would begin with "me" and a willingness to learn more about diet change, not dependence upon the medical community.

Before doing this fast I'd written a 6-page letter to the doctor I was about to see at Duke University Medical Center and explained all of my symptoms to her in great detail. She had access to a lot of information about me before I even went to see her for my appointment. When I did see this doctor at Duke she ran lots of blood tests on me. Everything came back fine.

She said, *"Danny, we can't tell from these tests you have rheumatoid arthritis, but we definitely know that you have arthritis."* Sometimes the tests show false-negatives. Apparently, there are about 150 different types of arthritis. Her recommendation to me was more drug prescriptions. Then she told me that nobody ever gets cured from arthritis. She said there is no cure for it and that I'd probably end up in a wheelchair.

I said to her, *"So you're telling me what all the other doctors have told me?"* She said, *"Yes."* I said, *"Thank you very much. But here are your drugs back. I'm going to come back in 3 months and prove to you that what we eat causes 90% of the physical problems we experience today. I'm going to prove this to you because I've been reading a lot of books and I found out that when I fasted for 5 days I was able to get rid of most of my arthritis pain. So it's food related. I know I'm onto something."*

"98 Percent of My Arthritis Was Gone"

I went back home and devoured more books. I wasn't afraid of the cost of buying a book anymore after having a $3,500 MRI, or paying the $250 one-time doctor visit that lasted under an hour. So I read and kept on reading until finding a reference to a mostly raw food diet often referred to as the Hallelujah diet. This led me to drive from New Bern to Shelby, North Carolina so I could attend a free seminar about it.

While at the seminar, I heard from literally dozens of people, including a few doctors and nurses still working in the medical community. Others were simply regular folks who had all types of physical problems go away after going on a mostly raw food diet. I heard stuff that was astounding. Things we've all heard there is no cure for had simply gone away as soon as the sick person changed their diet. Many of these people stated they had medical records to prove what they were saying too.

Some of the many diseases mentioned included things like cancer, arthritis, fibromyalgia, allergies, acid reflux, autism, ADD, high blood pressure and diabetes and many more. This greatly inspired me to start following this type of mostly raw diet.

I began attending the Hallelujah Diet Saturday seminars and culinary classes often, driving six hours each way. I made wonderful new friends and learned as much as I could from each one. I also started drinking fresh vegetable juices everyday, along with a green drink called BarleyMax.

During the first three months on this diet I lost 42 pounds and 98% of my arthritis was gone. When I walked into the appointment at Duke University Medical Center three months later for my follow-up visit the doctor didn't know who I was. She literally almost had tears in her eyes. She lit up like a light bulb and said, "*Danny, is that you?*" I said, "*Yes, ma'am.*" Then she asked, "*What have you done?*"

I sat her down for 30 minutes and told her the story. I told her I'd cut out all meat, caffeine, dairy products, white sugar and white flour from my diet. I explained about being a vegan and eating healthy living foods ... and that I juiced lots of vegetables and fruits daily. And I told her that I was consuming about 85% raw foods and 15% cooked vegetables.

Then I had this doctor raise my arms and squeeze my hands and feet. When she'd squeezed my feet three months earlier I almost jumped through the roof because of the pain. But now I told her to squeeze my joints as hard as she could. There wasn't even the slightest bit of pain. My doctor was completely amazed!

During this visit, I was also glad to point out how the smell under both armpits was gone. I told her I discovered that smell came from uric acid in my body, which had been produced to break down the large quantity of animal products I'd been consuming. But now my body had expelled this acid because I was no longer consuming animal based food products.

I shared with her that as the uric acid in my body declined the odor went away. I'd spoken to other people who'd experienced the same thing as me. After changing their diet, some of them would go to bed at night and wake up the next morning with their bed sheets yellow. Those yellow stains were from their body sweating out excess uric acid. While that didn't happen to me, I did talk to people who had the physical problems I'd had and experienced similar things.

After speaking with this doctor at Duke she almost had tears in her eyes. She said, "*Danny, you're doing the right thing. Only one other person I've ever spoken to has done what you've done and they had the same results. But you've blown that person away.*" She then said, "*I'm so proud of you. I'm on the same medications that I prescribed to you. I have arthritis in my hands, and I thought we just all get it from old age.*"

I said, "*No ma'am. It's a result of our diet. If you study some societies around the world there are instances where arthritis hardly exists -- if at all. The cause of my illness was what we refer to as the Standard American Diet.*"

After changing my diet, all of the physical problems that I'd been experiencing went away. Not only that, I look younger now too. People see me now and sometimes can't believe it's me. Some of the gray even went out of my hair, as it turned browner. My skin started to get a "glow" to it. I've had people who've asked me, "*What skin cream do you use for your face?*"

"The Right Foods Can Help Your Body Rebuild"

After 3 ½ years on a diet that was about 85% raw and 15% cooked vegetables, most of the arthritis went away, but not all of it. As of January 1st of this year (2009), I went totally raw in my diet. In other words, I'm currently on a 100% living foods vegan diet. For months now, I've noticed improvement in how I feel regarding the arthritis that was still bothering me. Just about all of the arthritic pain I ever had in my body is now completely gone.

I found I was eating more than 15% cooked foods. By going with 100% raw, it made it simpler for me to truly adapt to a living foods lifestyle. After going 100% raw I then found myself eating way too many nuts and seeds. So I'm still learning more each day.

I now enjoy unbelievably enormous amounts of energy and vitality … along with no more arthritis. My sleep is good and my thinking is also much clearer. I never get tired in the middle of the day or require a nap. My weight is now a normal 157 pounds at 5' 10" tall, down from 215 pounds. I love this healthy lifestyle and have learned, "*Nothing tastes as good as good health feels!*" Our health should be a priority. Many reach the prime of their lives and then have to spend all their savings trying to regain their health back.

For me, this diet wasn't so much of a choice as it was a necessity. In other words, I had to do the diet because I had to. If I hadn't been sick then I wouldn't have done the diet. But then I started to like it. Then I kept doing it because I loved it. And now I do it because it's my lifestyle. I would not go back now for nothing. The benefits of this lifestyle outweigh the enjoyment of the unhealthy foods I used to eat.

My dad told me once that if he were ever sick then he'd adopt this diet too. But since he wasn't sick he wasn't changing his diet. Recently, however, my dad went to the doctor and found out he had prostate cancer. He came to me and said, "*Well son, what do I need to do?*" So he started on a mostly raw diet.

Dad weighed 270 pounds when he began and now he's down to 210 pounds. He not only looks great but also says he has a lot more energy. His PSA levels have dropped over 2 points in 6 months.

"Your Body Craves Living Foods"

I'd ask anyone who is considering changing their diet to one that consists of mostly raw vegetables and fruits, "*What do you have to lose?*" The body is composed of living cells and needs living foods for nourishment. Foods that are cooked or canned or otherwise processed are "dead" foods. Your body craves living foods in order to be healthy.

In my opinion, the greatest thing that ever happened to me was getting sick with arthritis. I would've never gone this path unless I'd gotten sick. Adopting a plant-based diet was hard at the beginning. But since then, I've learned about thousands of varieties of vegetables and fruits … and how to prepare them.

Take onion bread for example. You can dehydrate it and make a sandwich with tomatoes, spinach and seeds with Italian herbs that even my father says is delicious.

And what about dessert? You can make a dairy-free treat that tastes like ice cream with frozen bananas or nuts and fresh blueberries. I've had all-natural, raw substitutes

137

that taste very much like chocolate, pudding, cakes, spaghetti and pizza ... all the foods I used to love in the past. I've just had to learn how to prepare these raw foods in a new way.

How many times have you seen people work on a hobby ... like car restoration or something? You see them putting incredible effort into making sure all the parts are right ... that it's polished properly ... and that the oil level is perfect, etc. Yet, when it comes to how they care for their own bodies, many of those same individuals would come up short.

My father and I now teach Biblical Nutrition 101 classes at church. The class has grown 300% and many have had wonderful healing testimonies since adopting a mostly 85% raw foods lifestyle. One gentleman in our class had to watch his son get married behind a glass enclosure because his asthma and allergies were so bad he could not breathe and had to wear a special machine around his neck to breathe. He came to class, learned what we learned, and both he and his wife adopted this lifestyle.

Within six weeks he no longer needed any medications - - nor the device he wore around his neck. He now has a normal life and his wife has had improvement in energy, sleep and weight loss. These are just a couple of the things we've seen in our class.

What an amazing journey this has been (and will be). A raw living foods diet and lifestyle can help a person be different than they are now. Everyone around you will see the changes. It's not easy, but anything worth having is worth working towards; and health is certainly a priority.

....

Danny Garris is owner of Garris TV in New Bern, North Carolina.

15
A Living Food Diet Overview

The following information is based upon the type of primarily raw plant-based diet most of those featured in this book used with great success. (An exception would be the Whole Food macrobiotic approach discussed in the chapter featuring the interview with Mariana Pina-Bergtold).

There are many opinions among raw food advocates about which raw food diet variation is best. While there is no way to know for sure what is "best" for every individual it seems like a good idea to begin following a plan that has produced many outstanding results for so many people.

An individual may begin seeing positive health results quickly (as little as a few weeks). For others, it will take several months. By simply taking harmful foods out of your diet, and replacing them with living raw foods, your immune system is given a chance to function as its highest levels and your body may begin to heal itself.

Raw "living" foods make up 80-85% of this diet. Cooked foods can make up 15-20% of the other portion. The basic approach is to primarily consume plant foods that contain living enzymes and the richest density of vitamins and minerals. The primary sources of these living foods are found within vegetables & fruits (including vegetable and fruit juices), nuts, seeds, certain oils, potatoes, squash, beans and a limited amount of grains.

Raw Vegetables (and Vegetable Juices)

Vegetables: Veggies offer you the greatest source of vitamins and minerals in raw form. Their varieties of color: green, red, yellow, orange and purple ... also suggest a variety of nutritional content within differing varieties. In general, you can eat as many raw vegetables as you want.

Fresh Raw Fruits: Fresh produce (organic if possible). Fruits offer the 2nd greatest amount of nutritional value to your body. Your diet cannot consist mostly or totally of fruit because fruits don't contain most of the nutrition your body needs. But they're great for breakfast, desserts and all natural snack treats such as smoothies and frozen sorbets.

Healthy Fats: If you're not going to eat meat then where can your body get needed fat content? From all-natural seeds, nuts, avocadoes, olives and other like sources. One well-known (and recommended) supplement is Flaxseed Oil.

Beverages: Pure Distilled Water, Fresh vegetable juices, fresh fruit juices. (Carrot juice is often used as a staple juice), caffeine-free teas, cereal-coffees, small amounts of bottled organic juices.

Cow Milk Substitutes: Nut butters, oat milk, rice milk, coconut milk, almond milk, and fruit creams made from blueberries, bananas and strawberries.

Grains: Oats, muesli, millet, granola, flaxseed, sprouted grains, whole grain cereals, whole grain breads, brown rice, etc.

Beans: Lima, kidney, black, navy, pinto, red, white, lentils, garbanzo, green, lentils, etc.

Nuts & Seeds: Raw walnuts, almonds, sunflower seeds, macadamia, etc.

Oils & Other Fats: Extra virgin Olive, Udo's Choice Blend, flaxseed, avocadoes, grapeseed, etc.

Seasonings: Celtic sea salt, dehydrated & fresh herbs, garlic, parsley, onions and other salt free seasonings.

Vegetable & Fruit Soups: Raw soups of all kinds.

Sweet Treats: Raw fruit pies, smoothies, dates, nuts, (toppings/sweeteners - raw honey, molasses, pure maple syrup, carob, rice syrup, stevia).

*B12 Supplement: Vegans (those who do not consume any meat or other animal products **MUST** supplement their diet with a B12 dietary supplement. There are several good ones on the market. A few will be recommended at **LivingFoodCures.com** in more detail.

Foods To Avoid:
All meat and other products derived from animals
Table salt
White Sugar
Dairy products
White Flour
Caffeine
Most processed food items packaged for long shelf life

"*What about the government's dietary recommendations and well-known food pyramid?*" you may ask. Whether you want to believe it or not, lobbyists have influenced virtually everything politicians and bureaucrats enact. Why should the "food pyramid" be any different?

There is no secret conspiracy here. The lobbying at Capitol Hill on behalf of food products is well documented. The government's food pyramid probably indicates which food manufacturers employ the most successful lobbyists. What science truly teaches about healthy eating isn't depicted by it.

16
An Interview with Jerrod Sessler
Testimony of Healing from Melanoma

I currently live with my family in Seattle, Washington. We're hoping to move to North Carolina in the near future. Right now, I balance business responsibilities with plenty of time to enjoy my 3 young kids and my beautiful wife, Nikki.

I'm known for being a NASCAR race driver, which I hope to do more of once we move. I am enjoying coaching my kids in kart racing for the time being. My main business is running a company I founded called HomeTask. We franchise a handyman brand called, "Yellow Van Handyman," and I'm working to grow that with current locations in sixteen states and in Canada. We also have another business called Freggies, which is a 100% organic produce delivery service that we started here in Seattle. We are planning to grow Freggies nationally as well.

In 1998 I went to see a doctor to get a checkup for NASCAR racing. I had an itchy mole on my back at the time, which the doctor looked at. He told me not to worry about it. But in 1999, about a year and a half later, my mom looked at it after becoming concerned at my habit of scratching my back on the corners of walls. The mole was irregularly shaped and had an irregular color to it. Those things are characteristics of melanoma, although we didn't realize it at the time.

My mom scheduled an appointment with the dermatologist and just by looking at it the doctor was pretty sure it was melanoma. I asked the doctor to cut the whole mole out instead of just taking a sample of it as she originally intended.

About a week afterwards, I was driving down the freeway and my sister called me. She was crying. She asked me if I'd talked to mom. I said, *"No."* And she said, *"Well, you need to call her and get to a doctor."* I knew at that moment - - at 29 yrs of age -- I'd just been diagnosed with cancer. From that day forward, many people that knew me treated me as though I was dying or already dead.

"Cancer in My Lymph Nodes"

There had been some delay in the diagnosis being communicated to my family because the doctor had been out of town for a few days. Being both a nurse, and an interested party though, my mother was able to help us finally get the results of the biopsy test.

It's hard to remember how I felt exactly upon hearing this news. I didn't know if I was going to be okay or not, but I believed God had a plan in all of this. My wife and I didn't have children at the time and I remember thinking, *"What is Nikki's life going to be like after my life ends? Is she going to be okay? Is she going to remarry? Is she going to live her dreams of having children?"*

I knew if I died I was going to heaven. But at the same time, I thought about the things I still wanted to do in this life. So those thoughts are something I had to wrestle with. I didn't know God was going to heal me. But once I began to realize the cause of disease I really started having confidence that I could see results within a healing process that had been successful for thousands of others. It was not standard medical protocol. No no, something much more mature, authentic and complete than the stab in the dark the common chemical treatments provide.

In my opinion, the fact I'd eaten chicken at least once a day for several years contributed to me getting cancer. I've

143

never been a big red meat, pork or fish eater, although I have had my share of each. I did, however, eat lots of chicken and turkey regularly. The chief issue with chicken and other animal products is the animal protein content, which Dr. T. Colin Campbell definitively describes in his book, "*The China Study.*" We can also consider the way chicken is produced today, which compounds the protein issue. In as short as five weeks, and with the help of a lot of chemicals, a chick can be slaughtered for dinner.

I now know that all of us have choices regarding our health. You can choose to put death on the end of your fork … and that's your choice. Or, you can choose to put life on the end of your fork … and that's a choice also. After the diagnosis, I began thinking of this each time I raised a fork to my mouth, "*Am I eating life or death?*"

Some of the doctors said my condition was stage-4 melanoma, which is very advanced, as there are only 5 stages. The melanoma grew deeper around a hair follicle, which caused the confusion in the determination of stage 3 versus stage 4. Some of the doctors said it was stage 3. The big problem, of course, is that they'd found evidence of cancer in my lymph nodes. And once cancer is found there then the fear is that it has potentially spread throughout the body.

Melanoma is known as the worst, fastest moving sort of cancer. When cancer gets into the bloodstream then melanoma often travels to high blood flow organs such as the liver, lungs and brain. This means a return diagnosis of melanoma is often quick … and deadly. What is happening on the skin may simply be a manifestation of what is happening somewhere else in the body.

The bottom line is that my prognosis, from a medical standpoint, was pretty grim. Most people who are diagnosed with what I was diagnosed with do not live very long. The doctors said I had a 40% chance of living another 5 years and a 5% chance of living another 10 years.

They said if I submitted to the standard medical treatment for this diagnosis (which included options for chemotherapy, radiation and interferon) then they felt it would improve my odds about 15%.

Those odds were not what I was looking for. I wanted to live a full life. I wanted a family. I wanted to continue driving racecars. So I started looking for something else.

"I Had to Find Out More About that Diet"

About a year or two before getting the cancer diagnosis, my wife and I had traveled to Chicago and spent a day with my aunt and uncle. They consumed a mostly raw food diet as taught by a health ministry called Hallelujah Acres.

My aunt had been diagnosed with Multiple Sclerosis about 20 years prior to changing her diet. As far as we could tell, she lived a fairly normal life. We didn't even know she had MS until we returned from the trip and I told my mom how "crazy" their diet was.

One of my first thoughts after discovering I had cancer was that I had to find out more about that diet so I could see if it could help me. One of the first pieces of information I got was a video called, *"How to Eliminate Sickness"* (now called: *"God's Way To Ultimate Health"*). In this video, Dr. George Malkmus talks about nutritional causes for diseases and things that need to be done in order to avoid them. (Visit www.hacres.com for more information about Hallelujah Acres).

We watched the video on Christmas Day, 1999, at my sister's house. I made a commitment that day to change my diet and lifestyle. While I did have some lymph nodes removed for testing a few days after I saw that video, I did not submit to any more medical procedures for my condition such as chemotherapy, radiation, drugs, double blind studies, interferon, etc.

Although my doctors eventually suggested the possibility of trying some experimental drugs, we ended up choosing to have the doctors simply "monitor" my situation for the time being. I wanted to see if the diet change would help me so we set up an appointment for a checkup 3 months later.

"The Physicians Were Amazed"

When I walked in for that appointment the physicians were amazed. They observed how I looked good because I'd lost some weight. They said my color looked good and that I appeared to be very healthy. We saw them again at the 6-month point and the reaction was the same. The doctor said we didn't need to return until the 12-month point. Again, we received the same response and so we were given leave for another full year. Our doctor told us in private that he believed in what we were doing but he was concerned I'd eventually go back to eating a Standard American Diet and the cancer would return.

I stayed with the diet though. Each time I went in for checkups I'd have to drink this nasty shake so they could see inside my body with a CAT scan. When I laid down on the table for the scans the machine injected me with something that felt really weird. After 2 years of this kind of monitoring I decided to end these appointments with the dermatologist.

I felt like I knew enough at that point to end the doctor's monitoring. I was also concerned about the injected chemicals and the shake they had me drink for these scans. That was the last time I've been to see a doctor.

After changing my diet, one of the first things I noticed was a difference in my energy level. I started feeling better right away. But there was a certain "clarity of mind" it brought also. It was as if a fog was lifted from my ability to think clearly. A friend of mine describes this phenomenon as being "scary clear." It's sort of like a heightened level of awareness of being.

Another area I noticed a change was with regards to my emotions. I started feeling like my self-control was radically heightened. I just felt more emotionally "level."

I also experienced dramatic results in weight loss. I'd had a little bit of a belly. I hadn't felt like I was in shape for a long time. But eating this new way eventually allowed me to shed 60 pounds. I hover now in the low 160s.

I don't really care what the scale says though. The important thing is how I feel. I've been working out more, lately, so my body fat is probably around 6% and I feel more toned now than ever before. If you've read "*Eat to Live*," by Dr. Joel Fuhrman, you'll see a weight chart in his book that I found to be pretty accurate as far as my own weight goes.

"So Much Food, So Little Time"

Changing my entire diet was hard to do at first. It was probably one of the hardest things I've ever had to do. The thing is … it's mainly mental. In the beginning, you think you've got to give up everything you now eat. But you need to get through that transition period to the point where you realize there is more freedom, flexibility and variety in a mostly raw vegan diet than what you've enjoyed up to this point in your life.

The flavor spectrum within a vegan diet is many times greater than what's found in a Standard American Diet. The variety of dishes you can make is amazing. You could literally try a new piece of produce everyday for the rest of your life and never repeat anything.

When you take all the different kinds of produce available out there and put them into new combinations then you've got unlimited variety. I've eaten more than

5,000 salads since changing my diet yet I've never eaten the same salad twice! How many dishes and combinations can you come up with for a thousand different kinds of vegetables, fruits, nuts, herbs, seeds, etc?

"Ten Years Later..."

As of this writing, I am nearly past the 10-year point with no indication of any physical ailment. My latest mantra this past year has been, "*So much food, so little time.*" There is so much food out there I want to try. But I'll never be able to experience it all.

My wife and I probably have 60 vegan recipe books on our shelf. We've collected thousands of recipes. I love being in the kitchen too. My mom brought me up in the kitchen. So I'd say about one-third of what we eat is stuff I've come up with by just going into the kitchen and creating something. I love doing that!

We also host a regular meet-up on Tuesday nights in our home. We make 3 or 4 new recipes each week, which totals up around 200 brand new recipes every year! I don't get excited about many of the dishes but this variety has enabled us to find some that we really love to eat and make!

I also speak at events locally, regionally and travel abroad to share my story and encourage people to take control over their lives by considering the things they eat and the impact those choices have on their existence. I can't imagine limiting myself to the Standard American Diet ever again.

"It Couldn't Be Better"

One of the things I can't stress enough is that there is a transition period that, for some, could last a lifetime. If you are interested in trying this then don't feel like you have to jump in with both feet the first day, week or month. There are a host of what I call transitional foods that are good to use as a stepping-stone between the Standard American Diet and a truly healthful one. If you want some direction in this, see my Facebook or web page.

The number one recommendation I'd make to anyone considering this kind of diet change is to not make a short-term commitment. Make a long-term commitment but remember you don't have to make radical changes overnight.

Make small changes with a focus. The only way you'll ever be able to make this a long-term change is to commit to educating yourself. Most of us view education as something for teens. We must get past this thinking and realize we are required to live a life of learning. If we stop learning we start dying.

You've got to commit to education. If you go into this for just a month then you'll probably not stay with it. Start with my book, *"5% Chance."* In it, you'll find recommendations for other books such as *"The China Study,"* and *"Eat to Live."* If you don't educate yourself then you will not grow. You will want to live the truth not because I have told it to you but because you have learned it for yourself and you are beginning to experience the reality of it in your own life.

We're all learning new things and being educated everyday. But what is the source of our learning? Is it coming from good books … or the latest advertisement on a billboard someplace?

Reading books that are full of truth will change how you think about food. So I'd encourage others to challenge themselves with regards to getting educated about food. The struggle here is having a good coach or curriculum to follow from a trusted source.

I would also require your source to be unmotivated by money. So, the key is getting good coaching. The reason is because the coach establishes the curriculum. The

149

curriculum in these terms includes the list of books that a coach would recommend.

Having a coach or a guide is much better than hitting the bookstore health section and getting lost in the pretty covers -- or worse -- misinformation some of these books contain. Visit my Facebook or web page for some free virtual coaching! My coach has been Hallelujah Acres and the teaching they put out. I trust them; have gotten to know them and they've never led me astray!

I understand why there are those who may be skeptical about the idea that diet can bring healing from a serious condition like cancer because I was one of them. When I was told many years ago I needed to be a vegan and avoid animal products to improve my health I thought it was crazy!

Our knowledge as individuals is limited. Even collectively, we only really know a small fraction of the total knowledge available. Because of that we need to be open to the possibility of being wrong. Education can help us overcome our ignorance in many areas. God is not cursed with ignorance as we are. He knows our condition and He is gracious with us.

You've got to try and approach most things in life with an open mind. If there is one thing we're missing in this culture it's an understanding of how much the messages we hear are centered on marketing. People who do nothing but try and figure out ways to get us to take money out of our wallet are marketing to us constantly.

The first few years I was on this diet I probably only ate about 50% raw. I still ate a lot of processed foods. There were a few times when I didn't drink enough water, or ate things that contained MSG or other excitotoxins. But I still lost weight. I still felt better.

I was also eating conventional produce until about the 4th year into the diet change. Then I started consuming largely organic produce. It took us several years to get out of eating any canned food products. For the first two years I was still eating French-fries from McDonald's about once a month. I did that until I didn't like the taste of them anymore.

Right now, I consume 90+% raw vegetables and fruits. The status of my health is great. It couldn't be better. I now feel as if the benefits of this lifestyle are endless.

…………………………

You can contact Jerrod on Facebook. Jerrod Sessler's various businesses, including those mentioned in this chapter, may be found at the following URLs:

www.HomeTask.com
 www.Freggies.com
www.hope4health.org
www.JerrodSessler.com
Twitter Jerrod: @Sessler

17
An Interview with
Samuel Ericsson
Testimony of Healing from Bladder Cancer

$\mathbf{M}$y wife, Bobby and I live in Harper's Ferry, West Virginia, near the Blue Ridge Mountains. I've worked as an attorney for 40 years.

I was a lawyer for over 10 years with a major law firm in Los Angeles. From there, I headed the Christian Legal Society for 10 years, which is a group of over 4,500 Christian lawyers and judges in Washington, D.C.

For the past 20 years I've led an organization called Advocates International, which is a global network that links lawyers from 150 countries. We encourage and work with lawyers internationally to do what they should be doing with regard to religious freedoms, human rights and conflict resolution. Throughout my career, I've been privileged to be involved with the Supreme Court in over 50 briefs dealing with 1st Amendment and Constitutional Law issues.

One of the ongoing challenges I face as a part of my job involves fundraising. This is the type of fundraising where I've had 30 to 40 people at a time completely dependent upon my ability to raise funds to keep international operations going. Since we're involved with human rights issues around the globe, funds need to be raised in order to keep up with the number of cases we're involved with.

There were times in the past when I'd put in 20-hour workdays. I didn't take care of myself in terms of getting proper rest. Even though I ate what I thought was a pretty healthy diet, I neglected to get proper rest and exercise. Those things, coupled with the high-stress naturally a part of my job, isn't good for the body. I believe those were the main reasons why I eventually got sick from cancer.

"Massive Amount of Cancer in My Bladder"

I found out I had cancer as a result of some physical problems I'd been experiencing. My doctor basically told me there was no medical hope for my recovery. Chemo, radiation, drugs and surgery are the standard tools a medical doctor uses to treat this disease. The oncologist told me that he'd found a massive amount of cancer in my bladder. I knew the medical tools he could offer me probably wouldn't be able to help much.

The doctor said, *"Sam, in a typical case of your kind of bladder cancer, if patients do chemo, radiation, drugs and surgery, then 60% of those patients will survive at least 5 years. But your cancer is 20 times worse than typical."* In other words, there was no doubt I was facing a real problem.

Upon hearing that news, my wife and I wanted to be open regarding treatment options. We decided that I'd try the best "medicine" could offer and the best "natural remedies" that could be applied. I chose to have certain cancerous growths removed from inside my body over the course of several surgeries. And I also opted to try a couple of different chemo treatments.

The surgeries, of course, never got to the root of the problem. All surgery can really do is remove the cell-growth caused by this disease. But if the cause is still there then the problems simply don't go away.

The first chemotherapy administered to me was called "BCG," a treatment that included live tuberculosis. It was applied as a wash into my bladder. That made me very sick. I came down with symptoms of TB almost immediately. I

153

sweated profusely at night, had cold chills and lost about 20 pounds after 5 weeks of treatments. The doctor finally said, "*I don't think this is working.*"

There was also another form of chemo the doctor wanted to try also. I wasn't keen on taking it, but he assured me I wouldn't get sick. After the first treatment, however, I developed a severe rash within 2 hours. So my body had very bad reactions to both attempts at trying chemotherapy.

"A Healthy Lifestyle"

I think one reason why the chemo treatments affected me like they did was because I was trying to build up my immune system. A healthy immune system is a main factor in good health. We need to build up our immune system and not do things to undermine it.

My wife Bobby has been very much into nutrition for over 30 years. She had read George Malkmus' book on diet and health. I then read it after being diagnosed. I thought his nutritional approach to health made sense so we both started on the diet he recommended.

Up to that point our diet had been pretty healthy compared to the typical Standard American Diet. We'd avoided fast foods and most junk foods for many years. We pretty much avoided red meats and ate only limited amounts of fish and poultry occasionally. My wife routinely ground her own grain and made fresh breads as well.

We'd also tried to avoid other unhealthy things such as white sugar and white flour -- which are nutritionally worthless. So we'd stayed away from many unhealthy things in our diet. But when I was diagnosed with cancer we decided to become even more committed to a lifestyle that included doing everything we could to eat healthy.

Had we heard about vegan diet programs before this? Yes, of course. We knew about veganism. We have friends who are 7th Day Adventists and they're vegans. We knew that Adventists who are vegans tend to be very healthy.

I now know that cancer is primarily caused by what we put into our bodies. If we don't eat the right things and choose to eat wrong things then the root cause of the sickness will never be addressed. The cancer will not go away until its cause is dealt with.

Bobby and I immediately began eliminating most of the other things we shouldn't be eating. We still had salmon for dinner on occasion. The conventional wisdom says that salmon is good for you. It wasn't until we discovered how much toxicity can be associated with domesticated salmon that we eliminated the fish from our diet too.

Both my wife and I began juicing every day. I probably juice about a ton of carrots a year now … about 5 pounds a day. That makes about a quart of carrot juice, which I drink 3 times throughout the day.

Another thing I immediately began doing was getting a proper night's rest. Instead of sleeping only 4 or 5 hours a night, I began going to bed at 9:30 pm and getting at least 7-8 hours of sleep.

There were some other changes we implemented too. Making time for exercise and getting out in the sun became important. Drinking pure water throughout the day also became a priority.

People need to know that getting healthy is much more than simply eating right. They need to have a healthy "lifestyle." You can have a good diet, but if you're not getting proper rest, exercise and sunlight along with reducing stress then everything may not come out rosy.

The biggest challenge for me has been trying to consistently implement this lifestyle into my work life. Since I'm the head of a global network that operates in over 150 countries, I'm still expected to travel to conferences and meetings all over the world.

Try juicing carrots if you're traveling in Nigeria, Kazakhstan or China. It's very difficult to follow this type of vegan lifestyle when traveling throughout certain parts of the world. Some may argue it's impossible to do if one lives in various countries because fresh fruits and vegetables may not be readily available.

One thing I had to do was reduce my traveling from around 125,000 miles to about 40,000 miles a year. I substantially reduced my international travel schedule because I had to.

When I do have to travel nowadays I take powdered vegetables with me, including carrot powder and BarleyMax. Even though they can't replace fresh vegetables for juicing they can be used to create relatively nutritious vegetable drinks.

I always try to eat salads when I'm on the road. It can be tough getting good salads in many places of the world though. There are times when the only salad I can get is a plate of iceberg lettuce, which isn't very nutritious. I just have to make do with what is available to me.

"Moving to a Plant-Based Diet"

After adapting a completely plant-based diet I quickly found that I had more energy. Another thing was losing weight. I'd been about 15-20 pounds overweight and the extra weight trimmed right off me. I slept better and began feeling better overall even though it was tough staying with the program 100%.

I'd go to my doctor for a checkup every few months and he'd scope me to look for new cancer. The few times he found some new cancer growth he'd suggest that I have it surgically removed. But even though I've had surgeries, one important thing about my cancer was that it had never become "rooted" in my organs. Even the large mass of cancerous growth in my bladder had never embedded itself into my interior muscles.

One reason why I think that was the case is because of the higher quality diet my wife had me on for years prior to all of this. That enabled my immune system to put up a pretty good fight against the cancer cells even after growths began forming in my body.

As of this moment, I'm still not what you'd call "cancer-free." Technically speaking, I still have some cancer in my body, and I go for regular monitoring. But I live a very active life and stay busy with my legal activities all around the world.

I was scoped just last November and the doctor found a bit of cancer in me. I know my body pretty well and one thing I've found is that if I eat things I shouldn't eat my body will let me know it right away.

To be honest, there were times when I consumed things that I knew weren't good for me. For example, I'd have coffee on occasion. And this past Christmas my dad sent me some Sees Candy for the holidays. I ate a few pieces of that chocolate. There were a few other things I also ate that I shouldn't have eaten. My bladder started bleeding profusely within 24 hours as a result.

Once again, I saw there are absolutely some things I shouldn't be eating because they're not good for me at all. If I had to rate my adherence to the new diet I'd probably give myself a "B." (My wife, however, would probably grade it "C+").

The main reason why I think I'm not completely free of cancer is because of my work. For example, 6 months ago our organization had a legal conference that brought together 1000 lawyers from 100 countries. I had to raise over a million dollars at the time. To pull off that kind of event in Washington adds a lot of stress to my life. Stress can be a huge factor with this particular disease.

Being involved with cultural issues, such as religious freedom and human rights on a regular basis, can also be very stressful. Right now, I have 22 people who depend on me to pay their salaries. I have to do a lot of ongoing fundraising. So I've still got a lot on my plate. My wife thinks this job-related stress is the main reason why the cancer is still hanging on. That's my excuse right now anyway.

On this point though, I feel as though Advocates International is very important. I'm committed to it. There is nobody to take my place at the moment. Though I have some stress on me that others don't have, I want to continue doing what I do as long as I'm able to do it.

There is no doubt in my mind I would've been dead 8 years ago if I hadn't found this lifestyle. When my doctor told me that 60% of patients normally survive 5 years, but that my case was 20 times worse than usual, I'm sure I'd already be dead unless I had changed the way I was eating.

The doctor said I had the largest cancerous mass he'd ever seen in a bladder. Incidentally, in Sweden they call bladder cancer the "lawyers' cancer." That is because lawyers there have the highest incidence (among any vocational occupation) of bladder cancer. Again, that is in large part because being a trial lawyer is a high stress job.

Being in a trial is like being in a war. It's not like being in a checkers game. It's like war ... and highly stressful.

I would recommend to anyone who is sick and wants to get healthy that there is simply no substitute for building up your immune system. To build a healthy immune system, you must eliminate stuff that is bad for you: white sugar, white flour, meat and dairy products.

A hundred years ago, most Americans consumed about 4 pounds of cheese a year. Now the average American eats around 40 pounds of cheese each year -- primarily because of pizza. That 40 pounds of cheese is basically like eating the equivalent of a 3-pound container of Crisco shortening every single month because cheese is about 70% fat. Imagine a mother feeding her kids a Crisco can of fat every month ... 12 months out of the year. Think about that!

Then there is the issue of white sugar. A hundred years ago, the average American probably only consumed about 5 pounds of sugar per year. Now the average American consumes somewhere in the neighborhood of 180 pounds of refined white sugar per year. Soda pop, cereals and other popular food products in our culture are filled with it.

So when you total up just the amount of fat and sugar most people consume today you come up with about 220 pounds of junk. If someone has a health problem they need to eliminate fat, sugar and other harmful things. Then they'll be able to feed their body living foods to build up their body's immune system.

Eating vegetables, fruits and grains builds up the immune system. We must "eat smart" as opposed to choosing "death by fork."

One of the reasons why Bobby and I chose this type of living foods diet approach to health is because a woman in our church had multiple sclerosis. She was in her mid-50s, on crutches and on her way to being in a wheelchair. The doctor had given her no hope. She changed her diet, however, and today she is in her mid-60s and could probably run a marathon. Even the brain lesions she had as a result of the MS, which the doctors said could never be cleared away, are all gone.

I've met people who had type-2 diabetes and got healthy within weeks, and sometimes even within days, of simply eliminating the wrong foods and eating the right ones. We've seen things like this happen again and again. Moving from an animal based-diet to a plant-based one can produce incredible health results.

"A Better Way of Living"

From a strictly medical standpoint the odds are that I should be dead. I've met hundreds of others who should've been dead a long time ago from the illnesses they had. But after moving from an animal-based diet to a plant-based diet they were healed.

I can give you the names of 25 former friends of mine who had cancer and followed the conventional routine of chemo, radiation and drugs and they're all dead. So I had to choose.

If you have a health problem, whether it's diabetes, cancer, heart disease, obesity or whatever the issue is, then try this type of lifestyle for 90 days. Purpose to just do it for 90 days and see how you feel and look afterwards. Test yourself.

If you haven't improved then maybe it's not for you. But I've never met a single person who honestly followed this kind of program - without cheating - who regrets doing it.

One thing I have to say though is that I never could've changed my lifestyle by myself. My wife is a phenomenal cook, loves to bake and is very disciplined. She has walked this journey with me for 10 years now and in many ways has done the program better than me.

We enjoy great meals together. But it takes time to prepare them. Whether one uses a vegan or macrobiotic approach to their diet it's very important to have family support. If you're trying to eat a salad when everyone else is eating steak and fries and consuming malts then it can be very discouraging. So it's very important for me to acknowledge my wife's support in this.

From the day I found out I had cancer I never asked, "*Why me?*" My response has always been that this health challenge can be a gift if I use it to address issues that should be addressed and then help others in a way I could never have helped by simply being a lawyer.

One reason why I believe God let me get cancer is because I've been able to steer hundreds ... and maybe thousands ... of people to a better way of living than if I'd just been a "healthy" lawyer. As a matter of fact, I've personally sent out 1,200 copies of George Malkmus' book to others in recent years.

I think I'm the individual who has purchased the most copies of his book since it's been published. If I didn't believe in this lifestyle would I personally spend $15,000 to give the book to friends? I try to put my money into what I personally advocate.

A couple of weeks ago my wife and I went on our second "vegan cruise" together. We were onboard a cruise ship with about 840 others who've chosen to eat healthy. There was a panel discussion with some of those in our group who had recovered from serious illnesses such as cancer and Crohn's disease after changing to a plant-based diet.

Some individuals shared how they had metastasized cancers throughout their body. For example, one person had battled pancreatic cancer. Another had fought kidney cancer. And another had been diagnosed with cancer in the spine. I heard story after story from individuals who were sent home to die by doctors because of those cancers. But they are well today.

. . . .

Samuel Ericsson is the founder and president of ADVOCATES INTERNATIONAL™, 8001 Braddock Road, Suite 300, Springfield, VA 22151-2110. More information can be found on their website: www.advocatesinternational.org
Samuel's email address is: samericsson@gmail.com
For even more details about Samuel's testimony of healing visit: http://www.advocatesinternational.org/resources/Newsltrs/news04/cancer.htm

18

Some Closing Thoughts About a Living Food Diet

Does Eating This Way Guarantee Health? No, it doesn't. We live in a world that is both wonderful and broken at the same time. Health and sickness coexist side-by-side. None of us wish it were so -- but it is.

Even those I've interviewed, who are now either recovering or are completely disease-free after changing their diet, would never claim that changing to a new diet "always" brings 100% healing 100% of the time. Any disease, especially those in advanced stages, would require time for the body's immune system to fight that disease.

Was poor diet a primary contributor to illness? If so, then going on a "living food diet" would still take time to help a body rejuvenate. That being said, I believe there is hope for multitudes of those who are now sick. They've never probed the depth of the possibilities when it comes to health through nutrition.

I've read a number of stories from individuals diagnosed with even late-stage illnesses who've experienced dramatic healing and recovery. So there is almost never a reason not to try a raw, living diet ... especially when fighting disease.

Check with your doctor. Ask him or her if consuming a living food diet along the lines described here will hurt you. Odds are it won't. The odds are even greater you'll reap significant health rewards in the long run.

The Importance of Exercise & Sunshine

You didn't think you were going to get away with not doing any exercise, did you? Seriously now, I'm not suggesting you have to start running 6 miles a day or lift weights. But even if you switch to a living foods diet you still need exercise to be healthy.

The goal is to change your whole lifestyle. Why wouldn't you want to enjoy an active healthy lifestyle after going through all the effort of changing the way you eat?

Buy an iPod (or other digital audio recorder) fill it with your favorite music or educational audio materials and go walking. Walk. Walk. Walk. Then walk some more. Get outside in the sun and walk as often as you can. Fill your mind with good thoughts, your lungs with fresh air and your body with good food.

If you can't walk or do any exercise right now then focus on the diet. When you begin feeling better then get outside. Experience the sunshine on your skin and go for long walks.

One of the interviews in this book is with Judy Livingstone, who had multiple sclerosis. She was one step away from going into a wheelchair. After being on a living foods diet for 4 months she felt well enough to go for a short walk down the driveway of her home. The next day she went a little further up the road. And now, 5 years later, Judy and her husband hiked up 6 mountains together inside their home State of Maine last year.

The Easiest Ways to Change Your Diet

The best way to change over to a healthy raw diet and lifestyle is to re-educate your thinking. In the beginning, you'll have to remind yourself on a daily basis regarding the food facts we've discussed.

Eating healthy will become even easier when you begin feeling better and receive positive results back from health tests conducted by your physicians. In other words, you should start seeing results and benefiting physically. When that happens your motivation to continue will grow.

One good way to begin is to clear out your refrigerator, freezer and pantry. Remove meats, dairy items and processed foods. Replace them with fresh fruits, vegetables, dried beans, lentils, brown rice, nuts and legumes, etc.

The next thing you'll want to do is buy some good raw food and vegan recipe books. Most are inexpensive. Eating healthy can taste very good and be very rewarding to your palate. Your new diet never has to be bland or boring. As a matter of fact, when you stop using standard table salt and white sugar as additives to your food you'll probably begin to "taste" the things you're eating in a whole new way.

If necessary, seek out a professional vegan food specialist and take part in some food preparation classes. It'll be fun. You'll also learn many exciting ways to prepare raw foods and cooked vegetables. You can make healthy eating an adventure to last a lifetime.

Most cravings for old unhealthy foods should disappear after time. Your appetite and desire for healthy foods should eventually replace unhealthy ones.

There is no better way to eat for vibrant health and healing. You won't have to count calories, buy expensive pre-packaged meals, or follow complicated formulas. Before you know it, eating a disease-fighting living foods diet will be a natural part of your life.

When you go to a party or other social gathering take your own pre-prepared food with you. If you know there will be a salad you can eat at your destination then all the better. But whether that's the case or not, you can always bring small containers of your own pre-prepared foods.

Tell your hosts you are on a special diet for health reasons and say nothing more. I'm not suggesting that you

164

be rude, but in the long run it really doesn't matter what anyone thinks about your eating habits. It's your health you're fighting for ... not theirs.

I would tell anyone to consult with his or her doctor first before doing any diet change. Just once have I ever heard from somebody who said their doctor advised them to stay away from eating raw vegetables because it would be "too hard on their bleeding colon." I suggested they ask their physician if they could juice raw vegetables for the time being instead. That would be one way they could begin their journey.

With these things in mind I encourage you to try out this "living foods lifestyle" for at least 30 days. See for yourself if you don't feel amazingly better. See if you don't have more energy and experience other marvels in your body.

Take it one day at a time. If you happen to make a bad food choice during the interim then don't beat yourself over the head with guilt. Just choose right foods next time around.

Keep going. Let one step lead to another. Enjoy your walks. As the old adage goes, *"Today is a gift -- which is why it's called the present."*

Living foods can help your body cure itself. You may be astonished at the results.

Get Your "Bonus Chapter" at the Following Web Address ...

A special bonus chapter interview to your Living Food Cures book has been added at **www.LivingFoodCures.com**. Please download it at no cost (it comes with this book). This interview features Julie Wilkins, who shared how she focused on nutrition after having surgery to remove melanoma skin cancer.

During my interview with Julie, she talked about how one can successfully approach a change in diet for health reasons. She also discussed how she shops for "living foods" in her area, along with some products she has found particularly helpful for meal preparation.

Julie is an example of how local raw and whole food enthusiasts can impact their local marketplace and chain supermarkets for the better.

Download your digital pdf copy of my interview with Julie at the following web address. Go to ...
www.LivingFoodCures.com/Book/BonusChapter.html
to receive your free copy now.

Endnotes

[1] The term "veganism," as used in this book, refers to a plant-based diet that also avoids the use of animal-based food products.

[2] Macrobiotics – "The theory or practice of promoting well-being and longevity, principally by means of a diet consisting chiefly of whole grains and beans." Source: http://www.answers.com/topic/macrobiotics

[3] Joel Fuhrman, MD, *Eat to Live,* (New York: NY: Little, Brown & Co, 2003), pp. 142-45.

[4] Source: http://www.cancer.org/downloads/STT/500809web.pdf

[5] Rowen Pfeiffer, D.C., cited by George Malkmus, *The Hallelujah Diet*, Destiny Image Publishers, Shippensburg, PA) pp. 73-74.

[6] Breslow, N., C.W. Chan, G. Dhom, et al. 1977. Latent carcinoma of prostrate at autopsy in seven areas. Int. J. Cancer 20: 680-88.

[7] T. Colin Campbell PhD, *The China Study* (Dallas, TX: Benbella Books, 2004).

[8] Joel Fuhrman, MD, quoted in George Malkmus, *The Hallelujah Diet* (Shippensburg, PA: Destiny Image Publishers, Inc, 2006), p. 74.

[9] Nelson, N.J. 1996. Is chemoprevention research overrated or underfunded? Primary Care & Cancer 16 (8): 29-30.

[10] Chang-Claude, J., and R. Frentzel-Beyme. 1993. Dietary and lifestyle determinants of mortality among German vegetarians. *Int. J. Epidemiol.* 22 (2): 228-36; Kahn, H.A, R.I. Phillips, D.A. Snowdon, and W. Choi. 1984. Association between reported diet and all cause mortality: twenty-one-year follow up on 27,530 adult Seventh-Day Adventists. *Am. J. Epidemiol.* 119: 775-87; Nestle, M. 1999. Animal v. plant food in human diets and health: is the historical record unequivocal? *Proc. Nutr. Soc.* 58 (2): 211-28.

[11] Dr. William Castelli, M.D., as quoted in Joel Fuhrman, MD, *Eat to Live*, (New York: NY: Little, Brown & Co, 2003), p. 75.

[12] Barnard, N.D., A. Nicholson, and J.L. Howard. 1995. The medical costs attributed to meat consumption. *Preventive Medicine* 24: 646-55; Segasothy, M., and P.A. Phillips. 1999. Vegetarian diet: panacea for modern lifestyle disease? *QJM 92* (9): 531-44.

[13] Kahn, H.A., op. cit. in 1984. Association between reported deit and all-cause morality. *J. Am. Epid.*, pp. 775-79.

[14] The term "iatrogenic" refers to a condition that has been inadvertently brought about by either medical procedures in relation to diagnosis, treatment, procedure, physicians or surgery.

[15] George Malkmus, *The Hallelujah Diet* (Shippensburg, PA: Destiny Image Publishers, Inc, 2006), p. 85.

[16] Robert Cialdini, *Influence: The Psychology of Persuasian* (William Morrow, New York, 1993), p. 219.

[17] Allopathic – "relating to or being a system of medicine that aims to combat disease by using remedies (as drugs or surgery) which produce effects that are

different from or incompatible with those of the disease being treated."
Source: http://www.merriam-webster.com/dictionary/allopathic
Naturopathy – "a system of treatment of disease that avoids drugs and surgery and emphasizes the use of natural agents (as air, water, and herbs) and physical means (as tissue manipulation and electrotherapy)."
Source: http://www.merriam-webster.com/medical/naturopathy
Natural Hygiene - "(Natural) Hygiene is that branch of biology which investigates the conditions upon which health and life depend, and the means by which they are sustained in their virtue and purity." Source: http://naturalhygienesociety.org/what_is_natural_hygiene.html

[18] For more on this comparison, see George Malkmus, *The Hallelujah Diet* (Shippensburg, PA: Destiny Image Publishers, Inc, 2006), p.111.
Also, see Dr Philip Chua's article entitled "*Vegetarian Diet and Longevity*," particularly his comments about A. D. Andrews, who wrote, *Fit Food For Men*. A.D. Andrews made an anatomical and structural comparison between carnivores and herbivores ... Source http://www.feu-nrmf.ph/drchua/pdf/V/VegetarianDietandLongevity.pdf
"Philip S. Chua, M.D. is Cardiac Surgeon Emeritus in Northwest Indiana, U.S.A., and currently the Chairman of Cardiovascular Surgery of the Cebu Cardiovascular Center, Cebu Doctors' Hospital, Cebu City, Philippines."
Source:http://www.cebudoctorsuniversity.edu/hospital/cardio/chua205.html

[19] Dr Neal Barnard, President of the Physicians Committee for Responsible Medicine, cited by George Malkmus, *The Hallelujah Diet*, Destiny Image Publishers, Shippensburg, PA) pps 67-68.

[20] George Malkmus, *The Hallelujah Diet*, Destiny Image Publishers, Shippensburg, PA) p. 119.

[21] Dr. Rowen Pfeifer, cited in George Malkmus, *The Hallelujah Diet*, Destiny Image Publishers, Shippensburg, PA) pp. 103-4.

[22] Maggi, S., J.L. Kelsey, J. Litvak and S.P. Hayes. 1991. Incidence of hip fractures in the elderly: a crossnational analysis. Osteoporosis Int. 1: 232-41.

[23] Francis M Pottenger, Jr., MD, Pottenger's Cats - A Study in Nutrition. Source: http://price-pottenger.org/Articles/PottsCats.html.

[24] George Malkmus, *The Hallelujah Diet*, Destiny Image Publishers, Shippensburg, PA) pp. 94-95.

Breinigsville, PA USA
14 October 2009
225783BV00003B/2/P